LIMITLESS

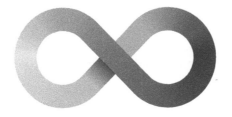

Unlock your hidden energy
and tap into the secrets
of peak performance

NICK POWELL

First published in Great Britain in 2019 by
Rethink Press (www.rethinkpress.com)

Cover image © Shutterstock|Anton Shahrai

The information, advice and suggestions in this book are provided by the author for informational purposes only and are not intended to replace medical care and advice. Use of the material set forth in the following pages is at the reader's discretion and is his or her sole responsibility. You should consult a professional healthcare practitioner before making any changes to your diet, exercise regime or lifestyle, especially if you have any health concerns, allergies, or are pregnant or breastfeeding. Neither the author nor the publisher should be held responsible for any injury, loss, damages or proceedings incurred in or associated in any way with the content of this book.

PRAISE

'This book represents practical advice and a user-friendly guide to biohacking, which is the art and science of improving our potential and whole quality of life. In my experience, once you apply the advice and new habits from *Limitless* you will feel at least a 50% increase in your energy levels and motivation. The only problem you may experience is that people won't believe you are so different by changing just a few inputs to your mind and body. Hopefully, more and more people will understand this causality and will contribute to our society and environment by living their real potential.'

DUŠAN PLICHTA, Founder & CEO, Powerlogy

'It's not often you come across a book packed with so much new and useful information. *Limitless* taught me about the importance of mitochondria and how you can adapt your lifestyle to put health first.'

HUTTON HENRY, CEO, Beyond M&A

'Nick's ability to take a complex topic such as body and brain performance and condense it down into an enjoyable, accessible and life-changing read is superb. If you're a high performing executive looking to supercharge your already high levels of energy and focus then this book is for you.'

SPENCER JOHN, Head of Investment Governance, Deutsche Bank

'*Limitless* is an enlightening book that offers some provocative, evidence-based approaches to anyone wanting to take back control of their health, energy and performance. If you want to learn more about the secrets of your mitochondria, a long health-span and staying younger than your biological years this is the book for you. And me.'

SARA MILNE ROWE, Performance Coach, Author and Speaker, Coaching Impact

'In *Limitless*, Nick brings together the latest thinking in micro-biology and positive psychology to create an easy-to-follow plan that will supercharge your energy levels and help you fulfil your true potential.'

JOSS DUGGAN, Entrepreneur, company builder and growth expert

'*Limitless* is a really accessible introduction to the world of bio-hacking tailored to the needs of busy executives and entre-preneurs. It covers a huge amount of ground and is therefore perfect for those who don't have the time to go hunting in the scientific literature and follow endless threads to get to action-able steps they can take to improve their own performance.'

MATT SMALLMAN, Founder

'I never thought I'd find myself drinking apple cider vinegar in a herbal tea on a Saturday night whilst trying to find local grass-fed beef on the internet but this book has opened my eyes entirely. The evidence is very well presented and sits neatly alongside helpful checklists to assist people in making better choices in an effort to take back control of our bodies.'

SEB ORTON, Partner of a leading law firm

CONTENTS

Foreword   1

Introduction   3

Why should you read this book?   3
Who is this book for?   4
My story   4
How to use this book   7
Where to find the recommended resources   8
What is biohacking?   8
Disclaimer   9

PART ONE: ENERGY, PERFORMANCE AND HEALTH-SPAN   11

One   It's all about your energy   13

Manage your energy and not your time   13
What are mitochondria?   15
The free radical theory, oxidative stress and
    inflammation   19
The link between mitochondria, energy,
    performance and health-span   23
Summary   24

Two   Can you live to 150?   27

Human lifespan   27
The other side of the coin   29
The future is coming   30
Do your research   32
Put yourself first   33
How to measure your age   36
Summary   37

PART TWO: TWELVE STRATEGIES FOR LIMITLESS ENERGY AND PEAK PERFORMANCE   **39**

Three   Eat what makes you feel great   **41**

Discover what is 'bad' for you   41
Eliminate foods for a month   43
What should you eat?   48
Not all 'good' foods are good for you   49
Miracle molecules   51
Summary   52

Four   Sleep quality trumps quantity   **57**

Why do you need to sleep?   57
How much sleep do you need?   59
Hacking sleep   61
Hacking jet lag   64
Summary   66

Five   What gets measured gets managed   **69**

Why track?   70
Core metrics – activity and sleep   70
Physical biometrics   73
Blood biomarkers   75
Hormone panel   78
Gut microbiome testing   79
DNA testing   80
Summary   81

Six   Burning fat for fuel   **83**

Fat is back   83
Ketosis   86
Why fasting is good for you   88
Intermittent fasting   90
Twenty-four-hour water fasting   92
Three-day water fasting   92
Summary   93

Seven   Move more and exercise less   **95**

Don't over-exercise   96
High-intensity interval training   98
Strength training   100
Get moving   102
Grounding   104
Summary   105

Eight   Embracing the magic of light   **109**

The wonders of light   110
Junk light   112
Irlen Syndrome   113
Is ultraviolet light bad for you?   115
Healing power of infrared light   116
Light and your day   118
Summary   120

Nine   Not all water is equal   **123**

Staying hydrated   123
Cellular hydration   125
Tap water   126
Water filters   129
Molecular hydrogen water   129
Drinking alcohol   131
Summary   133

Ten   Toxins will kill your performance   **135**

Toxins are a fact of life   135
Toxic mould   137
Pesticides   139
Cosmetics   141
EMFs   142
What else to watch out for?   144
Detoxification   145
Summary   146

Eleven   **Flood your body with oxygen**   **149**

Blood oxygen levels   149
Breathing correctly   150
Nasal breathing   153
Breathing techniques   153
Heart Rate Variability (HRV) training   155
Oxygen therapies   157
Summary   160

Twelve   **Getting cold makes you stronger**   **163**

Do you love the cold?   163
Taking a cold shower every day   167
Stepping it up   169
Summary   173

Thirteen   **Supplements are the last mile**   **175**

The last mile   175
The essentials   178
Timing and cycling your supplements   179
Intravenous (IV) vitamins   180
Nootropics, the smart drugs that work   180
Summary   185

Fourteen   **Hack your brain**   **187**

Meditation isn't woo   187
When you have a brainwave   190
Increasing alpha, theta and gamma brainwaves   192
Summary   199

PART THREE: BRINGING IT ALL TOGETHER   **203**

Fifteen   **How to make the strategies a habit**   **205**

Habits and routines   206
How to design a routine   207
Morning routines   208

Replacing bad habits with good habits   209
When your routine drops   211
Summary   212

Sixteen   Actionable checklists   **213**

If you do nothing else, do these   213
Starting out   214
Going further   218
Stepping it up a level   221

Seventeen   Real-world case studies   **225**

Matt   225
Tom   228
Paul   230
Simon   232

Conclusion   **235**

What's next?   236

Acknowledgements   **237**

The Author   **239**

This book is dedicated to my son, Rhys, who I'm sure will find this book an excellent resource for the rest of his long and happy life.

FOREWORD

What is one tip you would recommend for living with more energy, vitality and motivation?

This is a question I've asked all of my guests on Zestology podcast, which is my adventure to find more energy, vitality and motivation. It covers health tips, fun biohacking gadgets, supercharged supplements and some of the most respected and well-known experts on the planet.

When I ask that question, it's surprising how many of the answers centre around a few key themes. And those themes come up in *Limitless*.

My journey into the world of cutting-edge hacks for improving your health and energy began when I got ill in the jungle and had to have three months off work with post-viral fatigue. I spent a few months in bed, not knowing if I'd ever get back to normal. I tried everything to get back to normal. This book covers many strategies that I have personally implemented including fasting, red light exposure, hacking my sleep, supplementation, meditation, cold exposure and putting butter in my coffee. Sometimes it gets a little out of hand. For example, ever been tempted to spend a week in a dark room with electrodes stuck to your head? I did that recently (so you don't have to). It sounds weird, but was actually amazing, trust me.

Nick and I are part of the same tribe of biohackers/health tweakers/whatever you want to call us, and we strive to take our energy and performance to the next level. We both have a close relationship with Bulletproof®. I have interviewed founder Dave Asprey on a number of occasions and appeared on the Bulletproof® radio podcast and Nick is a certified Bulletproof® Coach. Nick has spent hundreds of hours learning the secrets of the world's top performers to understand how they hack their own biology to release massive amounts of untapped energy, enabling them to take their personal and business performance to the next level.

We live in challenging times, where there is so much pressure on our time and trying to find the right balance between work, spending quality time with our families, staying healthy, socialising with our friends and contributing to our community. Many people don't know what 'good' feels like. *Limitless* provides a holistic approach and will show you how to massively increase your energy levels through hacking your own biology.

I'm sure you'll enjoy this book and unlock your hidden energy to give you more vitality and motivation.

TONY WRIGHTON, TV presenter, author and
host of the Zestology podcast www.tonywrighton.com

Tony Wrighton is a familiar face on British TV as a sports presenter on Sky Sports. He's hosted lots of different sports on Sky Sports including football, golf, basketball, hockey, squash, pool, table tennis and even live ten-pin bowling. Tony is also a Master Practitioner and Trainer in NLP (Neuro-Linguistic Programming) and host of the popular podcast Zestology which has featured some of the biggest names in health, medicine, science and wellness worldwide.

INTRODUCTION

*Some people want it to happen, some wish
it would happen, others make it happen.*
MICHAEL JORDAN

Why should you read this book?

There are thousands of personal development books out there,
and you might be thinking, 'why is this one any different?' If you're
looking to find the key to operating in a high-performance state
and living a longer, healthier life, then you need to read this
book. *Limitless* breaks conventional wisdom and challenges
much of the well-known advice, providing you with a holistic
approach which will show you how to increase your energy,
performance and health-span through hacking your biology.

The world is a fantastic place, and you have more resources
at your disposal than ever before. You are living in a time of
abundance. On the flip side, you are living in a crazy world
of distraction, where your energy, time and attention are
under constant demand. You may struggle to balance time
between growing your career, time with family or friends,
going to the gym, life administration, cooking dinner and your
own self-care. Perhaps you feel that there never seems to be
enough hours in the day and you can rarely put yourself first.

Productivity tips and tricks won't make a step change in your
performance; energy management will always trump time
management. The advice provided by 'the experts' is heavily
influenced by big industry, much of which is making people

weaker and not stronger. You may think that you are highly energised but in reality you have forgotten what feeling 'great' is really like. How you feel right now is your new norm.

Limitless will open your eyes to a world of possibilities that you never knew existed and by following the strategies in this book you will massively increase your energy levels resulting in peak performance at home and at work.

You can take our Peak Performance Scorecard. It comprises forty questions to assess how well you are performing across all areas of your life: www.strongerself.global/scorecard.

Who is this book for?

This book is for you if, as I was three years ago, you are overweight, lacking energy and some of your spark. Do you feel your all-day energy is no longer there? Do you want to make the most of life? This book contains the vital ingredients that enabled me to put myself first and focus on my emotional, mental and physical performance.

The strategies outlined in this book apply to everybody, regardless of your job role, age, sex or background. This book is your gateway to the world of peak performance, biohacking, energy management and personal development.

Sit back, buckle up and keep an open mind.

My story

I was brought up in Port Talbot, a large industrial town in South Wales, United Kingdom. We lived on Sandfields Estate and next to a vast expense of sandy beach and it still brings a smile to my face whenever I think of it. 'The Estate', as it was more commonly known, was an earthy, grounded place with working-class people striving to provide for their families. I didn't have a poor upbringing, but it wasn't affluent. We didn't want for anything as my parents both worked incredibly hard which instilled an excellent work ethic in me.

My childhood was a happy one apart from a stammer which plagued me in my younger years and still trips me up now and again. I started to get tormented and bullied because of it, and it didn't help that my skin gains a suntan in minutes giving me a darker complexion and some racist nicknames. My parents decided to send me to Judo, to help me find the confidence to stand up to the bullies. I enjoyed Judo despite not winning a single fight until I was thirteen, but my perseverance prevailed, and I went on to become Welsh Champion when I was fifteen and was awarded my black belt when I was seventeen. Judo has been one of the biggest influences in my life.

I was academically strong and did well despite attending a dysfunctional school with a poor academic record. I went to Warwick University where I studied Electronic Engineering, and my father still says to this day that I cannot even wire a plug, and he's right. I graduated with a master's degree and secured a job in a management consultancy where I spent six years learning my trade. I then set up my own consultancy where I spent the next twelve years working with many large global businesses leading their business transformation programmes.

I've always had a strong work ethic and a fierce inner critic that has driven me to earn more money, be 'better' and more successful. As I got older, I found I couldn't work for as many hours as I could in my twenties; the all-day energy was no longer there. I was more stressed than at any other time in my life, and my priorities were skewed towards work first, followed by my family and then myself. At the time, I felt that it was just a part of getting older and that being a bit fat was part of the look of a forty-year-old. From the outside, my life appeared to be perfectly balanced and very successful, but it was tough trying to strike the right balance, and I couldn't focus and work as hard as I could when I was in my twenties. As the working week went on, it became more tiring. The weekends were used as downtime to help recharge for another relentless working week rather than spending quality time with my family.

I decided to take matters back into my own hands and delved deep into the world of peak performance to get more out of life, maximise my energy, reach my full potential, and turn back my biological clock. I found Bulletproof Coffee®, and this switched my brain on like nothing I had felt before. I then went on to focus on eating what makes me feel great and easily lost three stone of fat in just three months. Next, I experimented with optimising my sleep, meditation, cold therapy, light therapy and nootropics to further increase my energy and mental performance. My energy levels are now better than when I was in my early twenties, and my clarity of thought, cognitive abilities and decision making has never been better. Be prepared for the ripple effect because once people see your transformation they will start doing the same things.

As part of my journey, I certified as a Bulletproof® Coach with the Human Potential Institute and created Stronger Self®, to help high performing entrepreneurs and senior leaders to get even more out of life and re-establish balance by putting themselves first.

I now run a successful online community of people looking to improve their performance and live a higher quality of life. I also coach one to one with a select number of senior leaders and entrepreneurs to help them put themselves first, and in doing so, they make a step change in their overall performance across their professional and personal lives.

How to use this book

This book is in three parts:

Part One – *Energy, performance and health-span* focuses on the importance of energy management and why powering up your *mitochondria* is one of the most important things that you can do for your performance and health-expectancy. Part One also explores the question 'can you live to 150 years old?'.

Part Two – *Twelve strategies for limitless energy and peak performance* contains a series of focused chapters on how to biohack your way to limitless energy. Each chapter references leading scientific research from some of the world's leading doctors and is packed with actionable advice, top tips and case studies.

Part Three – *Bringing it all together* will show you how to put what you have learned into action, through the creation of habits that stick, become part of your daily routine and don't fall away. Part Three also includes a series of checklists to help consolidate what is covered in Part Two and a number of real-world case studies from my clients.

I recommend that you read the Introduction and Part One of this book because it sets some of the background and foundations for Part Two. However, when you get to Part Two, you have the option to either read the book chapter by chapter or jump around between chapters.

Where to find the recommended resources

I don't mention any specific products or further resources in this book because the world of biohacking, peak performance and personal development is moving at such a phenomenal pace. There is new scientific research, and new products are released every day, so by the time I complete this book, my recommended resources are likely to have changed.

Therefore, to keep this book current and provide you with the latest information, I've included a list of the recommended resources on the website: www.strongerself.global/limitless

Look out for the special indicators ® in this book which represent recommended resources associated with the text and go to the website above where the resources are listed by chapter.

The references in this book are also listed on this website for easy to access links.

What is biohacking?

Biohacking is an increasingly popular term that is creeping into the mainstream media. However, some people look a bit lost at the word and imagine you to be a biological terrorist. I like to describe it as taking control of your health and energy levels by harnessing the exciting intersection between biology, technology and your environment. It is a holistic approach to ensure your optimal physical, mental and emotional performance.

The word 'hacking' can give the impression of a quick fix or smart-cut, and while this is sometimes possible, quite often it takes hard work and dedication. I encourage you to listen to your body and do the things that make you feel great and ditch the things that don't. We are all different, so what may work for one person may not work for somebody else. I can't stress this point enough; do what works for you and keep an open mind.

In this book I introduce the term 'health-span'; you may not have come across it before. I like it as an alternative to longevity or life expectancy because it focuses on the quality of your life, i.e. how long are you going to live a healthy and disease-free life.

Disclaimer

I am not a medical doctor and therefore *will not and do not provide medical advice*, nor do I diagnose or treat disease. If you have any medical concerns or questions, then please consult a medical professional. On a serious note, do not start a new practice if you don't fully understand the implications and do check out a medical professional's opinion.

Although I'm a Bulletproof® Coach and certified by the Human Potential Institute, this book is in no way endorsed or linked to the Human Potential Institute or Bulletproof® or any of its subsidiaries.

ENERGY, PERFORMANCE AND HEALTH-SPAN

Part One of this book introduces how your body makes energy through the powerhouses of your cells and how free radicals, oxidative stress and inflammation impact your performance. It also asks the question: 'can we live to 150?'

CHAPTER ONE

IT'S ALL ABOUT YOUR ENERGY

Mitochondria is the powerhouse of the cell.
PHILIP SIEKEVITZ

In this chapter you will discover:

∞ Why managing your energy is more important than managing your time

∞ What mitochondria are and how your body makes energy

∞ Why mitochondria are so crucial to your energy, performance and health-span

∞ What free radicals are and how they lead to disease

∞ The link between mitochondria, your performance and your health-span

Manage your energy and not your time

To operate in a state of peak performance, you need to manage your energy first and then manage your time. I'm a big fan of time management techniques and productivity hacks and use them daily. However, many people place time management at the forefront of their personal development, and it's not the most important thing to manage.

When I refer to energy, I mean all-day energy, from the moment you wake up to the moment you go to bed. Avoiding slumps in your energy is the key to ensuring that you stay in a state of peak performance, deliver outstanding results and work consistently throughout the whole day.

If you're not running optimally and don't have energy, you could have all the tools, techniques and hacks available, but time will drift, you'll still procrastinate and not focus on the things that matter. If you get your energy levels right, then you'll have the resources to deploy effective time management techniques.

Your energy may be low if you are suffering from:

- ∞ Inability to focus resulting in procrastination and distraction

- ∞ Stress, tiredness and running on adrenaline

- ∞ Negative mood

- ∞ Poor motivation

- ∞ Using willpower to get things done

- ∞ Brain fog

- ∞ Making poor decisions

If you experience any of the above then you aren't putting yourself first, it's impacting your performance today, and it's likely to affect your long-term health. I'd like to ask you three questions:

∞ How do your energy levels feel right now?

∞ How would you score them from one to ten?

∞ How do your energy levels compare to when you were much younger?

Most of the energy your body produces is made by mitochondria, so if you want to increase your energy levels dramatically, then you need to understand how to protect your mitochondria and make them highly efficient. In the next section, I'm going to explain the basics of your mitochondria and why they are critically important to your energy, performance and health-span.

What are mitochondria?

Quite simply, without mitochondria, we would not exist.

The human body is made up of cells and according to an international team of researchers who published in 2013 in the 'Annals of Human Biology', there are about 37.2 trillion cells in the human body.[1] I can't even imagine that number of cells.

What if I then told you that most of the cells in your body contain at least one to two thousand mitochondria each and there is likely to be ten times this number in your brain, heart and ovaries (if you have them). This means that you're likely to have over seventy quadrillion (seventy thousand trillion) mitochondria in your body.

Mitochondria are tiny organelles (more on organelles later) that sit inside most of the cells in your body, and they are responsible for:

1. Energy production – they are called the powerhouse of our cells because they produce most of your energy from cellular respiration.

2. Cell death – they play a large part in determining when a cell will die through programmed cell death called apoptosis. Sometimes, cells don't die as they should do and can grow uncontrollably.

3. Specialised purpose – depending on the part of the body in which they are located, they may have a specific purpose, for example, mitochondria in the liver convert ammonia into a less toxic substance known as urea.

Mitochondria are critical to all life, and without them, we wouldn't exist. The performance of your mitochondria will determine how much energy you have, how you will perform in life and how long you are likely to live.

Figure 1 shows a graphical representation of what a single mitochondria (mitochondrion) looks like:

∞ Outer membrane – this is permeable and defines the shape of the mitochondria

∞ Inner-membrane – contains folds called cristae or spheres (a protein called $F_{0,}$ F_1 complexes) to increase the surface area and generate more energy

∞ Inter-membrane space – the volume between the outer and inner membranes

∞ Matrix – this is fluid in the inner-membrane that contains the mitochondrial DNA

∞ Mitochondrial DNA (mtDNA) – mitochondria have their own genetic material

∞ Ribosomes – to synthesise proteins

Figure 1 – diagram of a mitochondrion

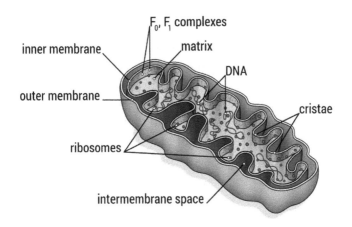

Your body makes energy either through anaerobic or aerobic respiration. Anaerobic respiration occurs in the absence of oxygen and takes place in the cytoplasm of the cells to provide a sudden burst of energy; whereas aerobic respiration occurs in the presence of oxygen and takes place inside the mito-chondria, producing over fifteen times more energy called adenosine triphosphate (ATP) than anaerobic respiration. ATP from aerobic respiration is created through a series of steps:

1. Glycolysis (using glucose) or beta-oxidisation (using fatty acids)

2. The Krebs cycle

3. Electron transport chain

Within mitochondria is the genetic material mtDNA, and magically this is only passed down by your mother. Sorry dads. The mtDNA is only passed down through the female egg because the sperm mtDNA is destroyed by the egg cell after fertilisation; and even if the mtDNA wasn't destroyed, there are 100,000 mitochondria in the human egg and only 100 in the sperm,[2] so the guys are outnumbered by the girls. The critical thing to note is that the natural strength of your mitochondria is linked to how healthy your mother and grandmother were before they conceived.

Remember I mentioned organelles earlier? I need to explain what they are. An organelle is a part of the cell that is located within the cell cytoplasm and plays a specialised function. Mitochondria are organelles, but they share very similar characteristics to bacteria as they:

1. Are a similar size (one to ten microns long) with a jellybean type shape

2. Divide in the same way

3. Have similar inner and outer membranes

4. Have their own DNA and synthesise their own proteins

Many scientists believe that mitochondria are derived from ancient bacteria and billions of years ago a symbiotic relationship formed between mitochondria and larger cells. This theory is called the endosymbiosis theory and was developed through the work of Lynn Margulis at Boston University in 1967.[3] Richard Dawkins, the British evolutionary biologist, quoted Lynn's work as:[4]

'I greatly admire Lynn Margulis's sheer courage and stamina in sticking by the endosymbiosis theory and carrying it through from being an unorthodoxy to an orthodoxy. I'm referring to the theory that the eukaryotic cell is a symbiotic union of primitive prokaryotic cells. This is one of the great achievements of twentieth-century evolutionary biology, and I greatly admire her for it.'

In effect, you have ancient bacteria living within the cells of your body that are responsible for providing energy to your cells, which means that you are more bacteria than you are human. Whether you believe the origins of mitochondria or not, one thing is for sure, they are the mechanism by which your body produces energy and without them you would not exist.

Mitochondria are sensitive to what you eat, toxins in your environment, your stress levels and even light. If you genuinely want to have a limitless amount of energy and extend your health-span, then you need to look after these little guys because they are the secret to you living a long and happy life.

If you would like to dig deeper into the science behind mitochondria, then I have shared additional reading in Resources Ⓡ.

The free radical theory, oxidative stress and inflammation

Molecules make up everything in nature from oxygen and amino acids to DNA and glucose. Stable molecules have electrons in pairs, and a molecule that doesn't have a pair of electrons is unstable and reactive. These unstable molecules are called free radicals and they travel through the body and steal an electron from another molecule to make themselves stable. In the process of doing this, they make the molecule that they stole from unstable. Excess free radicals are harmful because the chain reaction causes damage to DNA, cells and lipids, and is a significant contributor to ageing.

Free radicals can originate from a variety of sources, including:

1. Energy conversion – as part of aerobic respiration and specifically the electron transport chain, electrons can leak out to form free radicals.

2. The environment – what you eat, drink and the environment around you. This includes alcohol, tobacco smoke, pesticides and air pollutants.

3. Immune system – your body generates free radicals to fight off bacteria and viruses.

4. Chain reactions of free radicals – they go around stealing electrons from other molecules making them unstable and so the chain reaction continues.

When the mitochondria release a free radical, there is a risk that the free radical will damage the mitochondrial DNA, which is particularly susceptible to damage from free radicals because they aren't as well protected as the nuclear DNA. When the mitochondria get damaged through free radicals, their function reduces, and this leads to reduced energy output, an increase in free radical production and a decreased capability to buffer against free radicals. Also, remember that the mitochondria play a crucial role in signalling cell death through the process of apoptosis. If the mitochondria aren't working effectively, then this process is impaired, and it becomes a vicious cycle.

However, free radicals are required by your body, and they play a crucial role because your immune system will generate them to fight off bacteria and viruses. The critical point to understand is moderation. You want some free radicals in your body but not too many and indeed not left unchecked.

You're probably now wondering how your body keeps free radicals in check. It uses antioxidants to neutralise free radicals and to make enough antioxidants you need to eat a well-balanced diet high with a variety of plant-based foods.

If you think about a situation where the number of free radicals outnumbers the antioxidants, this is what is referred to as oxidative stress. When this occurs, the chain reaction I mentioned earlier goes into full swing and this is bad news because oxidative stress is an essential factor in many neuro-degenerative diseases[5] such as Alzheimer's, Parkinson's, Huntington's and amyotrophic lateral sclerosis (ALS). Oxidative stress is also linked to many chronic ailments[6] including cardio-vascular disease, stroke, heart attacks and cancer.

The diseases that originate from mitochondrial decline and oxidative stress start long before the symptoms of the disease manifest themselves, so it's essential that you start to look after your mitochondria now.

When your body is a under a heavy load of oxidative stress, you become inflamed, and this is a tell-tale sign that some-thing isn't right.

In summary:

excess free radicals = oxidative stress = inflammation in the body

It's critical that you manage any inflammation and avoid anything that makes you inflamed. How do you know if you suffer from inflammation?

You can monitor inflammation in a few different ways:

- ∞ Do you have any bloating in the stomach area? If you feel bloated, then you're inflamed and typically bloating in the stomach is as a result of eating or drinking something that doesn't agree with you.

- ∞ How has your weight fluctuated from yesterday? I weigh myself every single day, not because I'm obsessed about my weight, but I'm obsessed about what makes my weight fluctuate from one day to the next. For example, depending on what I've eaten my weight can be a whopping two kilograms heavier than the previous day.

- ∞ How is your brain feeling? Do you have any brain fog? You have ten times the mitochondria in your brain and therefore taking time to focus on how your brain feels will give you great insight into how much inflammation you may have.

- ∞ Measure inflammation in your body with a blood test and measure your high sensitivity C-reactive protein (hs-CRP) – see Chapter 5.

Mitochondria naturally decline with age, and when you're seventy, your mitochondria are running at significantly reduced efficiency compared to when you were thirty. Unsurprisingly, this is the focus of much anti-ageing work. When you make your mitochondria work more effectively, you will not only increase your energy and performance, but you will also slow down the ageing process.

The link between mitochondria, energy, performance and health-span

Now that you have a good understanding of mitochondria and how essential they are, can you see that your mitochondria directly impact your energy, performance and health-span?

If you power up your mitochondria then you are going to become highly energised, life becomes easier, your mood will change, and you will make smarter decisions. With more energy comes better performance in your career and more time at home. The secret to becoming a peak performer all rests with your mitochondria.

Powering up your mitochondria is also going to have a positive impact on your health because your cellular health is going to be rocking. By looking after your mitochondria, you're going to be looking after your entire body, and this is going to give you the best chance of living a long and disease-free life.

Health has three key dimensions: physical, mental, emotional; and all three must be carefully managed and put ahead of work and your family life. If you don't put yourself first, then you aren't going to be in the best position to help others.

When I meet a new client or generally chat to people about the work that I do with clients, I see a common theme. There is a genuine interest in performing better, having more energy and being healthier but when I start talking about living a much longer but healthier and disease-free life, the levels of excitement, intrigue and wonder go through the roof.

Most people want to live longer, and many don't think about dying. They push it to the back of their minds and focus on the day ahead. It scares the crap out of them to think about dying, those that they would leave behind, and not living their lives to the maximum.

Your mindset around how long you're going to live is an excellent indicator of how long you will live. A study conducted by Stanford University by Zahrt and Crum (2017)[7] covered 61,141 people in the USA and concluded that people's perceptions of their health plays an important role in their actual health outcomes.

Nobody wants to live a long life if it means losing their mind and being immobile, you want to have the mind and body of somebody who is much younger. This may seem like science fiction, and five to ten years ago it was. However, the good news is that there are now billions being spent on researching human health-span and I'm excited by it, especially for my son who will benefit from longevity science long after I've left this life.

Summary

In this chapter, you learned how critical mitochondria are to your ability to generate energy and if they aren't performing optimally then neither are you, physically, cognitively or emotionally. You also learned about free radicals, how they occur and the damage they can do to cells and your mitochondrial DNA. When there aren't enough antioxidants in the body to squash the free radicals, then oxidative stress and inflammation occurs, which leads to chronic diseases. How you perform in all aspects of your life directly relates to your mitochondria. If you look after them then your energy levels will massively increase, and you'll see improvements in all areas of your life.

References

1   Bianconi, E., Piovesan, A., Facchin, F., Beraudi A., Casadei, R., Frabetti F., Vitale L., Pelleri, M., Tassani, S., Piva, F., Perez-Amodio, S., Strippoli, P., & Canaider, S. (2013). An estimation of the number of cells in the human body. *Annals of Human Biology*, 40(6), 463–471. PMID: 23829164 – DOI: 10.3109/03014460.2013.807878

2   Ladoukakis E. D., & Eyre-Walker, A. (2004). "Evolutionary genetics: direct evidence of recombination in human mitochondrial DNA". *Heredity*, 93 (4), 321. PMID 15329668 – DOI:10.1038/SJ.HDY.6800572

3   Sagan, L. (1967). On the origin of mitosing cells. *Journal of Theoretical Biology*, 14(3), 225–274. PMID: 11541392 – DOI: 10.1016/0022-5193(67)90079-3

4   Brockman, J. (1995). *Gaia Is a Tough Bitch*. New York City: Simon & Schuster. Retrieved from www.edge.org/documents/ThirdCulture/n-Ch.7.html

5   Shukla, V., Mishra, S. K., & Pant, H. C. (2011). Oxidative stress in neurodegeneration. *Advances in pharmacological sciences, 2011, 572634*. PMID: 21941533 – DOI: 10.1155/2011/572634

6   Pham-Huy, L. A., He, H., & Pham-Huy, C. (2008). Free radicals, antioxidants in disease and health. *International Journal of Biomedical Science* (IJBS), 4(2), 89–96 PMID: 23675073 – Retrieved from www.ijbs.org/User/ContentFullText.aspx?VolumeNO=4&StartPage=89&Type=pdf

7   Zahrt, O. H., & Crum, A. J. (2017). Perceived physical activity and mortality: Evidence from three nationally representative US samples. *Health Psychology*, 36(11), 1017–1025. PMID: 28726475 – DOI: 10.1037/HEA0000531

CHAPTER TWO

CAN YOU LIVE TO 150?

The quality, not the longevity,
of one's life is what is important.
MARTIN LUTHER KING JR.

In this chapter you will discover:

∞ The journey and the future of human longevity

∞ If it's possible to live past 150

∞ Why you need to take responsibility for your health

∞ The technologies that aren't yet mainstream

Human lifespan

When the caveman existed, it's estimated that the average human lifespan was in the late twenties. Humans began having children at the age of thirteen and by the time they were twenty-six they were typically grandparents. Resources back then were scarce, and there was not enough to go around, so the grandparents wouldn't consume food and other resources that would otherwise have gone to their grandchildren. They typically died in their late twenties and so from an evolutionary point of view, humans were never meant to live past the age of thirty.

Over the past 150 years, we've been doing well to keep on increasing our lifespan each decade. We have moved on from a population that died through simple diseases in our early forties to a society that expects to live well into their seventies or eighties, and this is without doubt due to improvements in sanitation, agriculture and the control of diseases.

For the past 150 years, each generation has enjoyed a longer lifespan than its parents and grandparents, and I hope the trend continues despite concerns that the next generation may not live as long due to childhood obesity.

A study led by scientists from the Imperial College of London in collaboration with the World Health Organization predicted how life expectancy would change by 2030.[1]

The top five countries for life expectancy in 2030 are:

Men	Life expectancy at birth in 2010	Life expectancy at birth in 2030
South Korea	77.11	84.07
Australia	80.10	84.00
Switzerland	80.01	83.95
Canada	79.41	83.89
Netherlands	78.91	83.69

In the UK, male life expectancy will increase from 78.34 years in 2010 to 82.47 years in 2030 and in the USA, from 76.52 years in 2010 to 79.51 years in 2030.

Women	Life expectancy at birth in 2010	Life expectancy at birth in 2030
South Korea	84.23	90.82
France	84.86	88.55
Japan	86.66	88.41
Spain	84.83	88.07
Switzerland	84.59	87.70

In the UK, female life expectancy will increase from 82.32 years in 2010 to 85.25 years in 2030 and in the USA, women will increase from 81.24 years in 2010 to 83.32 years in 2030.

In *Resources* ® I have linked to the full table of results from the study.

The future looks rosy, but surely, we can do better than early to mid-eighties? The oldest person to ever live was Jeanne Calment of France, and she lived until she was 122 years old. So, we know that it's possible to live to 120, but why not longer? It's estimated that the longest living mammal, the bowhead whale, can live for over 200 years,[2] so there must be a biological reason why humans cannot live at least this long.

The other side of the coin

Although some reports state that life expectancy is set to increase, not everybody agrees. A report in 2005 in the New England Journal of Medicine calculated that in the first half of this century, life expectancy in the United States of America would level off or get shorter despite future advances in medical technology.[3]

The statistics show that human lifespan will continue to increase but what this doesn't reflect is the quality of the individual's life. Modern medicine can keep people alive longer but as it does, so does the risk of neurological diseases such as dementia, Parkinson's and Alzheimer's. The statistics are spiralling out of control:

∞ A 2018 report by Parkinson's UK estimates that Parkinson's diagnosis is likely to increase by almost 20% by 2025.[4]

∞ The World Alzheimer Report from 2018 estimates that there are currently 50 million people worldwide living with dementia and this number will more than triple to 152 million by 2050.[5]

∞ The International Agency for Research on Cancer, 'Cancer Tomorrow', estimates that worldwide, cancer is going to rise from eighteen million cases per year in 2018 to thirty million cases per year by 2040.[6]

∞ A 2017 report by researchers from King's College London predicts that the incidence of new strokes across Europe is likely to rise by 34% by 2035.[7]

Having a long lifespan is interesting but having a long health-span is what you need to aim for. I'm aiming to be much younger than my biological years.

The future is coming

It's not all bad because the ability to significantly increase our health-span and push the boundaries of what is possible is not that far away. Billions are being poured into extending the human health-span, anti-ageing technologies and the ability to rejuvenate the body. If you can stay healthy for the next twenty to thirty years, then there is a good chance that you could live a good quality of life into your hundreds.

In the next five years, there is going to be an explosion in technology, which is going to help prevent and treat some of the most life-threatening conditions. Here are two examples of technologies that are just around the corner and will dramatically increase our health-spans:

Stem cells

Stem cells are cells in your body that are abundant at birth and can change into any other cell in your body. As an adult, you have less stem cells but they can be extracted from your fat stores or bone marrow and injected into other parts of your body to help repair and rejuvenate. According to a 2017 report published by Grand View Research, Inc, the global stem cell industry is set to grow into a $15.63 billion-dollar industry by 2025.[8] It's now possible to have your baby's placenta frozen at birth ®, so their stem cells can be harvested if they need them later in life.

Genetic engineering (CRISPR)

CRISPR stands for 'Clustered Regularly Interspaced Short Palindromic Repeats' and enables the genes of cells to be edited. It's a controversial technique and highly regulated but is showing much promise for applications such as:

1. Editing the genetics of embryos to correct inherited errors that may cause disease

2. Destroying cancer where conventional treatment cannot

3. Developing new kinds of highly targeted pharmaceuticals

The world's billionaires are pouring their money into anti-ageing and longevity technology, so don't do anything stupid in the next twenty to thirty years and you'll have a great opportunity ahead of you. Aside from looking after your mitochondria, there are two principles to follow:

∞ Do your research

∞ Put yourself first

Do your research

The human population has exploded in growth over the past 200 years. In 1800 there were around 1 billion people, in 2011 there were 8 billion people, and based on a report by the United Nations in 2017, in 2050 there will be an estimated 9.8 billion people on Earth.[9] We are living longer than ever before, and this is putting enormous pressure on the global infrastructure, healthcare and the ability to produce high-quality food.

Food and pharmaceuticals are now multi-trillion-dollar industries and each time you watch TV or look at social media you are bombarded by advertisements, advice and scaremongering. History has told us not to believe the marketing drive from the 'Big Companies' which have pushed products as being healthy and it's now evident that some of them weren't.

'Big Pharma' is there to cure and not prevent disease. OK, they produce vaccinations, but most of their revenue comes from treating illnesses. I've heard too many stories in the UK where family and friends have visited their doctor, and they've used Google for help and been sent on their way with a prescription with no consideration for finding the root cause. I don't blame the doctors because they are chronically busy with limited time slots for each patient.

The point I'm making is that if you genuinely want to perform at your best and have a long health-span, then one of the most important things you can do is take responsibility for what you consume and expose yourself to. Many people have lost sight and consideration for what they consume and the impact it has on their bodies. Marketing dominates people, and they become brainwashed into two modes of thinking:

1. If they claim that it's healthy; then it must be

2. If I'm suffering symptoms, then the answer is to take some medicine rather than treat the root cause

There is one thing that I'm sure of, and that's if you want to perform at a high level and live a long health-span, you need to ignore all the marketing hype and do what is right for you. You are going to find a lot of conflicting opinions on the internet with lots of scientific studies thrown around from opposing sides. Do your research and work out what works for you. You are unique and not like anybody else on this planet, so what will work for you may not work for me. You will be uniquely sensitive to different things in your environment.

Also, when you have a specific medical complaint, please do your research so that you have all the right questions to ask your doctor and push hard until you find the root cause and get it addressed. If your doctor can't help you then seek out a Functional Medical Practitioner ®, whom you can work with to identify the root cause.

Put yourself first

When I work with my clients, I often ask them to think about how they should be prioritising their lives from the perspective of work, themselves and family. Friends could fall into the family category, and community interests could fall into the work category.

In most cases, the answer is:

Family, themselves, and then work

When I ask them how they are prioritising their lives, the answer is:

Work, family, and then themselves

Neither answer is correct. If you genuinely want to have beautiful relationships at home and put yourself in the best position to take your business and career to new heights, you need to become selfish and put yourself first.

Many clients shudder when I ask them to be selfish, so I always follow up with 'what's wrong with putting yourself first in the service of others?' It's a similar concept to what you've heard in the safety briefings on planes before take-off: *'When the oxygen mask drops down, please attach your mask before helping others.'*

CASE STUDY: Meet Matt. When I first started coaching Matt, he was struggling to focus, and his cognitive performance wasn't where he wanted it to be. He found it difficult to concentrate and was under immense pressure from a very demanding boss. His stress levels were high, and his work/life balance was deteriorating. Things weren't going well for Matt, and over a few weeks he had fallen off the rails, was burnt out and was partying hard which was further impacting his work/life balance. The result was overbearing work stress, and a meltdown at home.

Matt decided to focus on himself and build a handful of habits that would serve him well, help manage stress and set up every day for success. Within a few months Matt transformed his life and in doing so, he was able to rebuild his personal life and he secured a new role.

There is power in putting yourself first, and amazing things start to happen when you do so.

You need to look holistically at what is going on in your life and ensure you set yourself up for success, and by putting yourself first you're in the best place to serve others as a leader, a parent, a spouse and a friend.

CASE STUDY: Let me tell you about Dave. Dave was thirty-eight and working successfully as an independent management consultant, working with many global organisations delivering change programmes. He had built an excellent reputation and was always in demand for work. The problem was that Dave was overweight, suffering from low energy levels and was starting to struggle to focus in the afternoons and at the end of the week. He wasn't ill but didn't feel well, and the zing and sparkle were disappearing out of life, and he felt like he wasn't achieving his full potential. Dave worked hard during the week and then used the weekend to recover and wasn't fully present with his family. He thought this was normal and just a part of coming up to forty.

I am Dave, and I was wrong. There is no reason why you can't feel as great when you're forty or sixty as you did when you were twenty. You need to prioritise yourself, your energy levels and your health.

How to measure your age

You measure your age based on the number of years since you were born, but it's not a good indicator of how old you are. How often have you seen somebody and thought, crikey, they look great for their age, or conversely looked at somebody and said, 'they must have had a hard life'. Your age since birth is just a number and one that doesn't matter.

So how do you determine how old you are?

The truth is, you never truly know. Some tests can be performed to tell you your metabolic age or your telomere length, and these give an indication, but they have a margin of error and don't give you a complete picture. In the future, the convergence of microbiome analysis, DNA sequencing, blood testing and artificial intelligence has the best chance of giving your true biological age, but for now, it's best to focus on:

How do you feel?

Do you feel like you have a lot of energy, do you have aches and pains? How you feel is such a powerful indicator of your emotional, physical and mental health but it's a skill most people have lost because they never take the time to slow down and perform self-enquiry. They are too busy rushing from one thing to the next. Taking up a practice such as meditation enables you to tap into how you're feeling physically, mentally and emotionally and this is explained in Chapter 14.

How is your memory?

Is your memory starting to fail you, do you forget or misplace things easily? Are you able to learn and retain knowledge like you used to? There are ten times the mitochondria in your brain than anywhere else in your body, so your brain is a great indicator on how you're performing.

What are my biomarkers saying?

In Part Two of this book, there is a section in Chapter 5 which is dedicated to measuring your biological markers. There are a whole host of biomarkers that give you a good indication of how well you are performing. When you measure your biomarkers, it's an excellent point at which to act, and then you can track them over time. You can order most of these tests yourself and you can then work with a Functional Medical Practitioner if they flag any concerns.

Summary

We are all living longer, and it looks like the trend is projected to continue. More people are living into their hundreds than ever before, but as people are living longer, so the instances of neurodegenerative and chronic diseases are also increasing. If you wish to extend your health-span well into your hundreds and look and feel good, then you need to take control of your biology, do what is right for you and start putting yourself first. There is so much hype around emerging technologies such as blockchain, the rise of robots and artificial intelligence, but the big game changer is going to be at the intersection of biology and technology which is going to push the human health-span to new heights. The future is coming, and you need to hang on and not die of something silly in the meantime.

Can humans live to 150? It's not proven yet but with science moving at a fast pace with billions poured into health-span research, I'm banking on technological and biological innovation in the next twenty to thirty years to take me to one hundred and fifty.

References

1   Kontis, V., Bennett, J. E., Mathers, C. D., Li, G., Foreman, K., & Ezzati, M. (2017). Future life expectancy in 35 industrialised countries: projections with a Bayesian model ensemble. *The Lancet*, 389(10076), 1323–1335. PMID: 28236464 – DOI: 10.1016/S0140-6736(16)32381-9

2   Keane, M., Semeiks, J., Webb, A. E., Li, Y. I., Quesada, V., Craig, T., Madsen, L. B., van Dam, S., Brawand, D., Marques, P. I., Michalak, P., Kang, L., Bhak, J., Yim, H. S., Grishin, N. V., Nielsen, N. H., Heide-Jørgensen, M. P., Oziolor, E. M., Matson, C. W., Church, G. M., Stuart, G. W., Patton, J. C., George, J. C., Suydam, R., Larsen, K., López-Otín, C., O'Connell, M. J., Bickham, J. W., Thomsen, B., … de Magalhães, J. P. (2015). Insights into the evolution of longevity from the bowhead whale genome. *Cell reports*, 10(1), 112–22. PMID: 25565328 – DOI: 10.1016/J.CELREP.2014.12.008

3   Olshansky, S. J., Passaro, D. J., Hershow, R. C., Layden, J., Carnes, B. A., Brody, J., … & Ludwig, D. S. (2005). A potential decline in life expectancy in the United States in the 21st century. *New England Journal of Medicine*, 352(11), 1138–1145. PMID: 15784668 – DOI: 10.1056/NEJMSR043743

4   Parkinson's diagnoses set to increase by a fifth by 2025 (2018, January 08). Retrieved from www.parkinsons.org.uk/news/parkinsons-diagnoses-set-increase-fifth-2025

5   Patterson, C. (2018 September). World Alzheimer report 2018 – The state of the art of dementia research: New frontiers. Retrieved from www.alz.co.uk/research/WorldAlzheimerReport2018.pdf

6   World Health Organization. (2018). Cancer tomorrow. Retrieved from https://gco.iarc.fr/tomorrow/home

7   Stevens, E., Emmett, E., Wang, Y., McKevitt, C., & Wolfe, C. (2017). The burden of stroke in Europe. Retrieved from www.stroke.org.uk/sites/default/files/the_burden_of_stroke_in_europe_-_challenges_for_policy_makers.pdf

8   Stem Cell Market Size To Reach $15.63 Billion By 2025. (2017, June). Retrieved from www.grandviewresearch.com/press-release/global-stem-cells-market

9   Population Division World Population Prospects: The 2017 Revision. (2017). Retrieved from www.un.org/development/desa/publications/world-population-prospects-the-2017-revision.html

PART TWO

TWELVE STRATEGIES FOR LIMITLESS ENERGY AND PEAK PERFORMANCE

Part Two of this book introduces twelve strategies for powering up and protecting your mitochondria as well as reducing oxidative stress and inflammation. These strategies will help protect your ancient organelles, drastically increase your energy and performance and give you the best chance of a long and happy health-span.

CHAPTER THREE

EAT WHAT MAKES YOU FEEL GREAT

Let food be thy medicine and medicine be thy food.

HIPPOCRATES

In this chapter you will discover why:

- ∞ Diets are as taboo as religion, sex and politics

- ∞ Eating what makes you feel great is the best way to eat

- ∞ Eliminating suspect foods for a month will massively increase your energy levels

- ∞ Not all 'good' foods are good for you, so you need to listen to your body

Remember to look out for the recommended resources symbol ®.

Discover what is 'bad' for you

What you eat and drink each day is essential to your energy levels and how you will perform. I come from a background in systems implementation, so I can relate to the analogy 'rubbish in, rubbish out'. What you eat and drink is directly linked to how your body makes energy in your mitochondria.

A rule of thumb that many people use when hosting a dinner party is never to discuss religion, politics or sex. I'd like to add nutrition because it's become as taboo as sex, politics and religion. There are so many different types of diets including vegetarian, vegan, low carb, paleo, ketogenic and 5:2; there is too much debate on what works and what doesn't.

MYTH: **There is one universal diet that works for most people.**

TRUTH: What works for you, won't work for me because we are each unique. We will metabolise macronutrients differently, we are sensitive to different foods, and our gut microbiomes will respond better to some foods than others.

If you are focusing on what you eat and drink, then the chances are you're already in the top 5% of healthy people, and please don't think of it as a diet but as your unique lifestyle.

Listen to your body during and after you eat because all the information you could need is already there; you just aren't looking for it. You need to eat what makes you feel great, and if after a meal you don't feel fantastic and highly energised, there was something in your last meal that you shouldn't have eaten. If you have eaten something your body doesn't like, then you are likely to experience bloating in the stomach, brain fog and fatigue. If before and after you have eaten you record your pulse, it can help you to understand if you have eaten something that you may be sensitive to because your heart rate will increase by more than sixteen beats per minute. It's best to check your heart rate every 15 minutes.

Something to also consider is that if you are eating the same meal as your partner each evening, then it's likely that one of you will be eating something that doesn't suit them.

> **CASE STUDY:** John knew he had issues with wheat but refused to admit it to himself. When I asked him to notice how he felt after each time he ate, he quickly realised that when he ate wheat he didn't respond well, he felt bloated and lethargic, and this isn't how he wanted to feel. By correlating how he felt to what he ate, he was able to change his diet and avoid the foods that took away his energy.

Eliminate foods for a month

The following are a list of foods that you should eliminate from your diet for four weeks and assess how you feel each day by journaling. Consuming many of these foods can contribute to mitochondrial dysfunction and inflammation.

Sugar

What is it? There are over one hundred different names for sugar but look out for these common ones: anhydrous dextrose, brown sugar, cane sugar, corn sweetener, corn syrup, dextrose, evaporated cane juice, fructose sweetener, fruit juice concentrates, high-fructose corn syrup, honey, malt syrup, molasses, raw sugar, syrup and white sugar.

Where do you find it? Sugar hides in many foods, especially ones that you wouldn't think would have sugar, such as wholemeal bread, breakfast cereals and fruit juice.

Why avoid it? It will spike your insulin, giving you an energy high followed by an energy crash. Excessive sugar consumption is linked to type 2 diabetes,[1] cancer,[2] Alzheimer's,[3] cardiovascular disease[4] and liver disease.[5]

Alternatives: Starchy carbs such as sweet potato and healthy fats such as avocados, coconut oil, low mercury fatty fish and grass-fed, grass-finished meat.

Grains

What is it? Grains are divided into two subgroups; refined grains and whole grains. Refined grains start out as whole grains and they are then processed to give them a longer shelf life.

Where do you find it? Grains are in many foods and include wheat, rye, barley, oats, corn, millet and even gluten-free powders.

Why avoid it? There are many reasons why you should consider cutting out grains:

1. Grains contain high levels of phytic acid which can prevent you from absorbing some nutrients

2. Grains are often sprayed with a herbicide called glyphosate, which in 2015 was classified by the World Health Organization as a 'probable carcinogenic to humans'[6]

3. Grains can also cause high levels of inflammation[7]

4. Grains are also prone to mould (mycotoxins)[8]

Alternatives: Long grain white rice is a clean source of carbohydrates as it's pure starch. It contains few nutrients, but it also has a low toxin load. Don't consider gluten-free products because they often contain substitutes that are no better for you than gluten.

Dairy

What is it? Dairy products are derived from cattle.

Where do you find it? Cheese, milk, ice cream and desserts.

Why avoid it? Until 10,000 years ago we hadn't domesticated animals, and therefore never drank milk, and our bodies aren't designed to digest milk after the age of five. Dairy typically contains two types of proteins called beta-casein (A1 and A2). A1 beta-casein is difficult for humans to process and is inflammatory.[9] Dairy also stimulates the production of IGF1 (insulin growth like factor) which is associated with acne, breast cancer and prostate cancer.[10]

Alternatives: Goat's milk, sheep's milk and camel's milk (all have none or lower amounts of A1 beta-casein).

MYTH: **Margarine is good for you**

TRUTH: No, it's not. Margarine used to have high levels of trans-fats and these are the worst kind of fats that you could eat. Thankfully, it now contains trace amounts of trans-fats, but is still a highly processed food which turns liquid vegetable oils into solid fat.

Soy

What is it? Soybeans are legumes that originated in East Asia and are now grown all over the world. Soybeans are known as a superfood and are high in protein.

Where do you find it? Soy milk, tofu, various meat substitutes, soybean oil and soy protein.

Why avoid it?

1. Over 80%[11] of the world's Soybeans are produced by the USA, Brazil and Argentina and over 94%[12] of it is genetically modified and sprayed with glyphosate, which the World Health Organization says is likely to be carcinogenic.[6] Always go organic with Soybeans.

2. Soy contains significant amounts of isoflavones, which can activate oestrogen receptors in the body. For some people, isoflavones may impact their thyroid function.

3. Soy has been linked to a decrease in male fertility.[13]

Alternatives: Beans, nuts, seeds and mushrooms.

Vegetable oils and nut oils

What is it? I need to start with what this isn't. It's not olive oil, which is incredibly good for you (but don't cook with it because it oxidises at low heat). Vegetable oils have become a trendy alternative to saturated fats, but the process they go through to create the vegetable oil often includes pressing and heating highly toxic chemicals and solvents. It's just not food.

Where do you find it? Canola, corn, cottonseed, peanut, sunflower and soybean.

Why avoid it? There are numerous reasons to give vegetable oils a miss because they are:

1. Genetically modified, so are often sprayed with glyphosate.

2. Unstable and readily oxidise when cooking.

3. High in omega-6, which is linked to higher amounts of free radicals and oxidative stress.[14] The ratio of omega-6 to omega-3 in our diets should be around 4:1, and for most people, it's 16:1.

Alternatives: Olive oil, coconut oil, ghee and butter.

Artificial sweeteners

What is it? Artificial sweeteners are popular as an alternative to sugar.

Where do you find it? It's found in low sugar drinks and low-calorie foods. Most commonly known as aspartame, sucralose and acesulfame potassium.

Why avoid it? The internet is waging war on artificial sweeteners and whether they are 'good' or 'bad'. My take on this is that they are artificial and therefore not something people should be putting inside their bodies. Studies have linked artificial sweeteners with:

1. Cancer[15]

2. A 67% increase in the risk for diabetes[16]

3. Liver inflammation[17]

Alternatives: Water and flavoured water with lemon or lime.

It would be best if you avoided all processed food and that's not easy to do because it is everywhere. Processed food has a high toxin load, contains high amounts of sugar and contains damaged fats. In the category of processed foods, I would also include factory farmed, grain-fed meat and farmed fish because of their high toxic load.

By removing these foods from your diet, you will feel incredible and your energy levels will massively increase. Whenever I mistakenly re-introduce any of the above foods, it results in inflammation, brain fog and fatigue.

Remember to always eat what makes you feel great.

> **EXERCISE: Noticing how you feel.**
>
> The next meal you eat, take some time after the meal to notice how you feel.
>
> How is your cognition? Do you feel sharp or do you have brain fog?
>
> How do you feel physically? Do you have any signs of bloating?
>
> How energised are you? Do you feel strong or weak?

What should you eat?

Plant-based diets have gained in popularity, and the vegan movement is growing and shows no sign of slowing down. I'm a big advocate of an organic plant-based diet, and it's my view that most of your plate should be vegetables.

The war on meat has quite rightly pointed out that factory farmed animal products are linked with inflammation and therefore a whole host of chronic diseases. If I had to pick between factory farmed meat and a vegan diet, I would always go vegan. However, not all meat-based products are equal, and high-quality red meat that is grass-fed, and grass-finished is an excellent source of amino acids, collagen, vitamin B12 and omega 3 fatty acids. I'm not advocating a high protein Atkins-style diet because too much protein isn't good for your body but having a small to moderate amount of high-quality animal protein is good for you.

Having a diet that is rich in organic vegetables and high-quality animal protein is vital, but also, you need to consider:

1.   Healthy fats, such as coconut oil, avocados, eggs, pasture-raised meat, wild salmon and olive oil (don't cook with it)

2.   Starchy carbohydrates such as sweet potatoes and long grain white rice

Not all 'good' foods are good for you

Eating lots of green vegetables and different coloured vegetables is vital for a well-rounded and healthy diet and consuming this every day is important, primarily to absorb enough polyphenols. It's far better to consume high-quality foods as the nutrients and vitamins are more bio-available than in supplement form.

In the last section, soya was on the list of foods to avoid, and this may have come as a surprise. However, there are other fruit and vegetables that some people have an adverse reaction to and become inflamed. Therefore, I advise you to eat what makes you feel great and notice what foods don't.

I become inflamed and bloated whenever I eat any fruit and vegetables that are part of the nightshade family ⓡ, and these include ashwagandha, aubergines, tomatoes, peppers (bell peppers, chilli peppers, paprika, tamales, tomatillos, pimentos, cayenne) and potatoes.

Some of the above foods are more commonly known as superfoods, but unfortunately for me, they aren't. For some people (one in four), if they eat a nightshade fruit or vegetable it can result in:

∞ Irritable bowel disorders

∞ Heartburn

∞ Joint pain and sensitive nerves

∞ Autoimmune conditions

CASE STUDY: Simon started focusing on foods that were giving him energy versus the foods that took away his energy. As part of this exercise, the usual suspect foods had a negative impact on his performance, but there were also a few surprises. Simon noticed that when he ate pistachio nuts, he would have an energy crash a little later in the day. However, pistachio nuts are meant to be a superfood and are packed with nutrients and antioxidants. The problem that Simon was experiencing was due to mycotoxins in the pistachios because they can quite often be subject to mould problems.

The critical thing to remember is to notice what you eat and if you feel amazing after your meal then great but if you don't there is something in the meal you shouldn't have eaten.

Miracle molecules

There are two amazing molecules that you can only get from your food that have amazing benefits. There are supplements on the market that claim to contain these molecules, but they are nowhere near as impactful as getting them from your food. I'm sure that as science progresses, they will find a way to create supplements but for now, get them naturally. These miracle molecules are sulforaphane and polyphenols.

Sulforaphane is a molecule found in cruciferous vegetables. It is derived from glucoraphanin and is produced when it meets the enzyme myrosinase. When you chop or chew the plant, it starts the production of sulforaphane.

Sulforaphane is an immune stimulant and is also anti-inflammatory. It has been well studied and not only helps with a wide range of conditions but also acts as a protector:

∞ Increasing glutathione production[18]

∞ Supporting a healthy heart[19]

∞ Improving cognitive performance[20]

∞ Reducing the risk of cardiovascular disease[21]

∞ Helping to create cancer-fighting compounds[22]

∞ Improving liver function[23]

Sulforaphane comes from cruciferous vegetables, which include: bok choy, broccoli, Brussels sprouts, cabbage, cauliflower, collard greens, kale, mustard greens, radish, rocket and watercress. The best source of sulforaphane is broccoli sprouts (not Brussels sprouts) because they contain between ten and one hundred times more sulforaphane than mature broccoli. You can buy seeds and growing kits at home ®, and within a few days, you will have delicious broccoli sprouts to put on your salad.

Polyphenols ® are amazing molecules and are a type of antioxidant. You will generally find that most foods that are high in polyphenols have a slightly bitter taste to them. The highest concentration of polyphenols is found in blackcurrants, blueberries, coffee, dark chocolate, dark green vegetables, fresh and dried herbs, green tea, olives, pomegranates, red cabbage, red onion and red wine.

There are many benefits to consuming a wide range of polyphenols, and these are highlighted in a 2016 study[24] that looked at the positive role that polyphenols play in reducing oxidative stress and inflammation. The study found that polyphenols have beneficial properties which reduce inflammation, protect against cancer, protect against neurodegenerative diseases and lower the risk of cardiovascular disease.

Summary

Diets are fads, but a lifestyle change is permanent and regardless of what your dietary preference is, if you're focusing on what you eat then you're already on the right track. However, most people have never considered how they feel after they eat, and their new norm can include bloatedness, brain fog and energy crashes after they eat. When you start noticing how you feel after you eat and eliminate the foods that make you feel weak, you'll suddenly have a lot more energy, improve your health-span and increase your overall performance.

Your actions:

∞ Take the time after each meal and snack to make a note of how you feel. If you don't feel great, ie low energy, brain flog or bloating then question what was in the food

∞ Commit for a month to eliminate the foods in this chapter and see how you feel

∞ Find a local source and purchase:

~ Grass-fed, grass-finished meat ®

~ Organic vegetables ®

~ Wild-caught fish ®

∞ Grow your broccoli seeds at home for sulforaphane ®

∞ Bring more foods into your diet that are high in polyphenols ®

Part 3 of this book brings all the actions together in an easy-to-follow checklist.

References

1   Basu, S., Yoffe, P., Hills, N., & Lustig, R. H. (2013). The relationship of sugar to population-level diabetes prevalence: an econometric analysis of repeated cross-sectional data. PloS one, 8(2), e57873. PMID: 23460912 – DOI: 10.1103/PHYSREVLETT.119.211801

2   Jiang, Y., Pan, Y., Rhea, P. R., Tan, L., Gagea, M., Cohen, L., & Yang, P. (2016). A sucrose-enriched diet promotes tumorigenesis in mammary gland in part through the 12-lipoxygenase pathway. Cancer research, 76(1), 24–29. PMID: 26729790 – DOI: 10.1158/0008-5472.CAN-14-3432

3   Zheng, F., Yan, L., Yang, Z., Zhong, B., & Xie, W. (2018). HbA 1c, diabetes and cognitive decline: the English Longitudinal Study of Ageing. Diabetologia, 61(4), 839–848. PMID: 29368156 – DOI: 10.1007/S00125-017-4541-7

4   Yang, Q., Zhang, Z., Gregg, E. W., Flanders, W. D., Merritt, R., & Hu, F. B. (2014). Added sugar intake and cardiovascular diseases mortality among US adults. JAMA internal medicine, 174(4), 516–524. PMID: 24493081 – DOI: 10.1001/JAMAINTERNMED.2013.13563

5   Jensen, T., Abdelmalek, M. F., Sullivan, S., Nadeau, K. J. Green, M., Roncal, C., & Tolan, D. R. (2018). Fructose and sugar: a major mediator of non-alcoholic fatty liver disease. Journal of hepatology, 68(5), 1063–1075. PMID: 29408694 – DOI: 10.1016/J.JHEP.2018.01.019

6   Evaluation of five organophosphate insecticides and herbicides. (2015, March 20). Retrieved from: www.iarc.fr/wp-content/uploads/2018/07/MonographVolume112-1.pdf

7   De Punder, K., & Pruimboom, L. (2013). The dietary intake of wheat and other cereal grains and their role in inflammation. Nutrients, 5(3), 771–787. PMID: 23482055 – DOI:10.3390/NU5030771

8   Alshannaq, A., & Yu, J. H. (2017). Occurrence, Toxicity, and Analysis of Major Mycotoxins in Food. International journal of environmental research and public health, 14(6), 632. PMID: 28608841 – DOI: 10.3390/IJERPH14060632

9   Jianqin, S., Leiming, X., Lu, X., Yelland, G. W., Ni, J., & Clarke, A. J. (2015). Effects of milk containing only A2 beta casein versus milk containing both A1 and A2 beta casein proteins on gastrointestinal physiology, symptoms of discomfort, and cognitive behavior of people with self-reported intolerance to traditional cows' milk. Nutrition journal, 15, 35. PMID: 27039383 – DOI: 10.1186/S12937-016-0147-Z

10 Danby, W. (2009). Acne, dairy and cancer: The 5α-P link. Dermato-endocrinology, 1(1), 12–16. PMID: 20046583 – DOI:10.4161/DERM.1.1.7124

11 Statista (2018). Retrieved from: www.statista.com/statistics/263926/soybean-production-in-selected-countries-since-1980/

12   ISAAA (2017). Global Status of Commercialized Biotech/GM Crops in 2017: Biotech Crop Adoption Surges as Economic Benefits Accumulate in 22 Years. ISAAA Brief No. 53. Retrieved from: www.isaaa.org/resources/publications/briefs/53/download/isaaa-brief-53-2017.pdf

13   Chavarro, J. E., Toth, T. L., Sadio, S. M., & Hauser, R. (2008). Soy food and isoflavone intake in relation to semen quality parameters among men from an infertility clinic. *Human reproduction*, 23(11), 2584–2590. PMID: 18650557 – DOI: 10.1093/HUMREP/DEN243

14   Patterson, E., Wall, R., Fitzgerald, G. F., Ross, R. P., & Stanton, C. (2012). Health implications of high dietary omega-6 polyunsaturated fatty acids. *Journal of nutrition and metabolism*, 2012, 539426. PMID: 22570770 – DOI: 10.1155/2012/539426

15   Soffritti, M., Padovani, M., Tibaldi, E., Falcioni, L., Manservisi, F., & Belpoggi, F. (2014). The carcinogenic effects of aspartame: The urgent need for regulatory re-evaluation. *American journal of industrial medicine*, 57(4), 383–397. PMID: 24436139 – DOI: 10.1002/AJIM.22296

16   Nettleton, J. A., Lutsey, P. L., Wang, Y., Lima, J. A., Michos, E. D., & Jacobs, D. R. (2009). Diet soda intake and risk of incident metabolic syndrome and type 2 diabetes in the multi-ethnic study of atherosclerosis. *Diabetes care*, 32(4), 688–94. PMID: 19151203 – DOI: 10.2337/DC08-1799

17   Bian, X., Chi, L., Gao, B., Tu, P., Ru, H., & Lu, K. (2017). Gut microbiome response to sucralose and its potential role in inducing liver inflammation in mice. *Frontiers in physiology*, 8, 487 – PMID: 28790923 – DOI: 10.3389/FPHYS.2017.00487

18   Steele, M. L., Fuller, S., Patel, M., Kersaitis, C., Ooi, L., & Münch, G. (2013). Effect of Nrf2 activators on release of glutathione, cysteinylglycine and homocysteine by human U373 astroglial cells. *Redox biology*, 1(1), 441–5. PMID: 24191238 – DOI: 10.1016/J.REDOX.2013.08.006

19   Bai, Y., Wang, X., Zhao, S., Ma, C., Cui, J., & Zheng, Y. (2015). Sulforaphane protects against cardiovascular disease via Nrf2 activation. *Oxidative medicine and cellular longevity*, 2015, 407580. PMID: 26583056 – DOI: 10.1155/2015/407580

20   Dash, P. K., Zhao, J., Orsi, S. A., Zhang, M., & Moore, A. N. (2009). Sulforaphane improves cognitive function administered following traumatic brain injury. *Neuroscience letters*, 460(2), 103–107. PMID: 19515491 – DOI: 10.1016/J.NEULET.2009.04.028

21   Mirmiran, P., Bahadoran, Z., Hosseinpanah, Rajab, A., Asghari, A., & Azizi, F. (2012). Broccoli sprouts powder could improve serum triglyceride and oxidized LDL/LDL-cholesterol ratio in type 2 diabetic patients: A randomized double-blind placebo-controlled clinical trial. *Diabetes research and clinical practice*, 96(3), 348–354. PMID: 22325157 – DOI: 10.1016/J.DIABRES.2012.01.009

22   Zhang, Y., Talalay, P., Cho, C. G., & Posner, G. H. (1992). A major inducer of anticarcinogenic protective enzymes from broccoli: isolation and elucidation of structure. *Proceedings of the national academy of sciences*, 89(6), 2399–2403 PMID: 1549603

23   Oguz, A., Kapan, M., Kaplan, I., Alabalik, U., Ulger, B. V., Uslukaya, O., & Polat, Y. (2015). The effects of sulforaphane on the liver and remote organ damage in hepatic ischemia-reperfusion model formed with pringle maneuver in rats. *International Journal of Surgery*, 18, 163–168. PMID: 25924817 – DOI: 10.1016/J.IJSU.2015.04.049

24   Hussain, T., Tan, B., Yin, Y., Blachier, F., Tossou, M. C., & Rahu, N. (2016). Oxidative Stress and Inflammation: What Polyphenols Can Do for Us?. *Oxidative medicine and cellular longevity*, 2016, 7432797. PMID: 27738491 – DOI: 10.1155/2016/7432797

CHAPTER FOUR

SLEEP QUALITY TRUMPS QUANTITY

*Early to bed and early to rise makes
a man healthy, wealthy, and wise.*

BENJAMIN FRANKLIN

In this chapter you will discover:

- ∞ The link between circadian rhythms, sleep and your hormones

- ∞ How to work out how much sleep you need each night

- ∞ The easy ways to hack your sleep so that you improve the quality of your sleep

- ∞ How to handle jet lag so you can land from a flight and still perform

Remember to look out for the recommended resources symbol ⓡ.

Why do you need to sleep?

Sleep is a critical element of performing well, and you will feel great after a good night's sleep. You need to sleep to repair your body, process emotions and move short-term memories to your longer-term memory and if you don't get enough quality sleep, then you're going to impact your energy, performance and health-span. A lack of quality sleep is linked to many chronic conditions including high rates of cancer and stroke,[1] increased risk of obesity,[2] depression,[3] and diabetes.[4]

You are encoded with a circadian rhythm, which is often referred to as your 'body clock' or 'internal clock'. The word 'circadian' comes from the Latin words meaning 'about a day' and is roughly a twenty-four-hour cycle that follows the sun and controls your body's mechanisms, signalling for you to release critical hormones at specific times of the day, such as melatonin, cortisol, thyroid stimulating hormone and prolactin.

Understanding your circadian rhythms will help you to determine how late you should stay up and how early you should rise to do your best work. Each of our circadian rhythms is different; our bodies all operate to their unique rhythms, and this is called your chronotype. Your chronotype will, for instance, indicate if you do your best work in the morning or the evening. To find out your chronotype, you can either take an online test ®, or if you have had your DNA sequenced then you can work out your chronotype from there, but it's not easy because there are potentially twenty-two genetic variants associated with your chronotype.

How much sleep do you need?

When you sleep you go through cycles and each cycle will last about ninety minutes. Depending on how long you sleep you may have between four and six cycles per night. As part of the ninety-minute cycle you will go through four different phases of sleep:

∞ Phase 1 – very light sleep – a state when you're drifting off to sleep.

∞ Phase 2 – light sleep – where you spend most of your light sleep, and it prepares your body for the transition into deep sleep.

∞ Phase 3 – deep sleep – this is the most restorative and rejuvenating sleep stage and is where your body is in repair mode. When in a deep sleep, your heart and breathing rates regulate, your blood pressure drops, and your muscles are relaxed. In this phase, you are difficult to wake up.

∞ Phase 4 – REM (rapid eye movement sleep) – is your dream state and where your body processes emotions and moves short-term memories into your long-term memory.

While not strictly a sleep stage, it's also worth noting your awake time. Awake time is not just the time you spent awake at night; it also includes how long it took you to fall asleep once in bed.

Let's say you have five sleep cycles at night; you should expect that each sleep cycle will contain a differing amount of light, deep and REM sleep. For example:

Cycle 1–2 – more light and deep sleep

Cycle 3–5 – more REM sleep

A common question I get asked is 'how much sleep do I need each night?', and the answer isn't simple because it's unique to you and your chronotype. The standard eight hours a night blanket guideline has been debunked, the largest sleep study[5] ever conducted on 1.1 million people shows that the optimum amount of sleep each night is 6.5 hours. The same study revealed that the group that was sleeping eight hours a night were 12% more likely to die within a six-year period.

Remember that the ninety-minute sleep cycle is only an approximation so if you regularly sleep seven hours a night then it could mean that you have an eighty-four-minute sleep cycle.

> **EXERCISE: Calculating your ideal amount of sleep.**
>
> How long do you usually spend asleep at night in minutes?
>
> (Eg if you spend seven hours in bed a night this equates to 7 * 60 minutes = 420 minutes)
>
> Divide that number by 90 to get an approximation of how many sleep cycles you are currently having a night.
>
> (Eg 420 minutes/90 = 4.7 cycles)
>
> Round your number up to get a complete number of sleep cycles.
>
> (Eg five sleep cycles)
>
> Multiply the number of sleep cycles by 90 minutes.
>
> (Eg 5 * 90 minutes = 450 minutes = 7.5 hours)

What time do you want to wake up?

(Eg, let's say this is 6:30am, so your bedtime will be 11:00pm, in bed and sleeping)

Ensure you give yourself enough time to get to bed and set your alarm for 6:30am. The challenge is to wake up before your alarm goes off.

The ninety-minute sleep cycle is an approximation, and each person will vary slightly, so if you wake up way ahead of your alarm then move your bedtime later by fifteen minutes. If you sleep through your alarm, then move your bedtime earlier by fifteen minutes.

Focusing on your sleep cycles and therefore the quality of your sleep is far more important than focusing on your quantity of sleep. If you can wake up at the end of your ninety-minute sleep cycle, then you will awake refreshed and full of energy.

Hacking sleep

To hack your sleep, you first need to be able to track it, and when you start to monitor your sleep, you'll be able to draw conclusions about what you've done that day and how well you have slept. This will take a little time because there will be many variables at play, but you will start to notice a pattern and what makes an impact on your sleep.

It's also important to not get overly hung up on the quantity of sleep and what are the right ratios of REM, deep and light sleep. The first place to start is to purchase a device that measures both the quality and quantity of your sleep ®.

MYTH: **Snoring is harmless, and everybody does it.**

TRUTH: It may appear harmless to you, but your partner may have something to say about your snoring. Snoring can be a strong indicator of sleep apnea, and if untreated it can sap your energy and lead to significant health issues such as heart attack, diabetes and depression.[6]

If you move away from focusing on the quantity of your sleep and focus on the quality of your sleep, you'll benefit far more regarding your performance, and you may even be able to cut down the amount of sleep you need. Imagine what you could do with an additional one and a half hours a day?

Here are some strategies to improve the quality of your sleep:

∞ Don't drink any caffeine after 2pm – caffeine is a stimulant and will interfere with the quality of your sleep even if you think it doesn't. I'm always amazed at the number of people who will have an espresso after dinner and then complain that they can't sleep at night. Make the time earlier than 2pm if you are particularly sensitive to caffeine.

∞ Sleep in a cave – make sure the room is completely dark. Invest in some blackout curtains and tape up ® any LEDs on devices in your bedroom, especially if they are blue. It must be pitch black. Your brain and skin are sensitive to light, and this confuses your circadian rhythm leading to restless sleep.

∞ Alcohol – keep alcohol to a minimum because it will disturb your sleep. I find even having two glasses of wine can reduce my sleep score by ten points.

∞ Keep the room cool Ⓡ – aim for the temperature in the bedroom to be 18.5° Celsius. Nobody likes being too hot in bed, go for a cold room.

∞ Create a bedtime routine – this includes avoiding all electronic devices at least one hour before bedtime because the stimulation before going to sleep will stop you from falling asleep quickly and will limit your deep sleep.

∞ If you need to work late – install a screen filter on your computer Ⓡ to help block out the blue light and if you want to take this to the next level, invest in a pair of blue-blocking glasses. Ⓡ

∞ Take a magnesium supplement – most people are deficient in magnesium because they can't get it from food sources due to mass farming methods. Supplementing this mineral can make significant improvements in the quality of sleep. I take 400 to 500 mg before bed. Ⓡ

∞ Watch your exercise at night – for some people, if they exercise within two hours of their bedtime, it increases their adrenaline levels, heart rate, and body temperature, making it difficult to fall asleep.

∞ Get to bed before 11pm – because of your circadian rhythm, if you are awake after this time your cortisol level rises and you'll get a second wind.

∞ Honey, tea and apple cider vinegar – combine two
   tablespoons of apple cider vinegar and one tablespoon
   of honey and stir these into one cup of decaffeinated
   tea. This pre-bed cocktail will knock you out.
   It's worth the funky taste.[7]

∞ Write a journal for ten minutes before going to
   bed – to empty your head and stop yourself from
   overthinking as you try and drift off to sleep.

∞ EMFs – don't put your phone by your bed and sleep
   with it all night by your head. Put your phone on the
   other side of the room.

> **CASE STUDY:** Tom was complaining that he was waking
> up at 4am each morning and then couldn't get back to
> sleep. He was going through a lot at the time with a
> divorce and a new business, so there was a lot of stress
> in his life. When he woke up, he had so much spinning
> around his head he couldn't get back to sleep. It had
> been this way for a couple of years. Tom started taking
> magnesium at night and suddenly, he started sleeping
> through to 6am in the morning.

Hacking jet lag

Jet lag is something that I've battled with for some time. While
some trips have been bearable, there have been several
occasions when it's been very painful with little sleep. I've
flown transatlantic many times and faced different challenges
when flying east and west.

Flying east, I find it difficult to sleep on the flight. As I'm 6 feet 2 inches, sleeping in business class is difficult, and in economy, it's next to impossible. When I land, I'm sleep deprived and can't function for most of the day. If I take a nap, I find that it ruins my sleep patterns for the next two or three days.

Flying west, I work during the whole flight and stay up as late as I can, but despite trying many things, I always wake up between 3 and 4am and can't get back to sleep. I wake up so refreshed and wide awake. It's an 'oh, NO' moment, 'I'm awake now', then I crash and burn later in the afternoon.

I've now developed a tried and tested method to beat jet lag, even when flying in economy.

You will need to pack the following:

1. Noise-cancelling headphones ®

2. Blue-blocking glasses ®

3. LED earbuds to send light signals to your brain ®

4. Protein-based snacks ®

On the flight:

∞ Don't drink any alcohol; it will make you dehydrated and groggy when you land. There is nothing worse than stepping off an aeroplane and having a mild hangover kick in.

∞ Please don't eat the plane food; I've not come across anything edible even when travelling in business class. It's disgusting so eat before you fly and take the opportunity to fast on the flight (Chapter 6).

∞ Make sure you drink plenty of water to get well hydrated, aim to drink at least 300ml every hour you're on the plane.

∞ Use your noise-cancelling headphones to block out the noise of the aircraft; you'll be amazed at how loud the plane is. This noise is draining for your brain as it acts like static.

∞ Use blue-blocking glasses to help you fall asleep.

After the flight:

∞ If you land any time after lunchtime, avoid the temptation to have a nap. If you need to nap, try to have no more than ninety minutes (one sleep cycle).

∞ If it's sunny, get outside and get some sunlight, to help reset your circadian rhythm. If it's not sunny, then use LED ear buds to amplify the signal to your brain that it's daylight.

∞ Ground yourself to release static by going for a walk outside in your bare feet. It connects you with the ground, helps to reset your circadian rhythms and helps to discharge static that has built up in your body.

∞ Supplement with PQQ/CoQ10 Ⓡ to give your mitochondria a boost.

Summary

The importance of having enough sleep each night is critical, and I'm sure you've experienced poor performance when you haven't slept well. The link between getting enough sleep and your energy and health-span is well established, so if you do want to be at the top of your game then you need to focus on your sleep. The amount of sleep you need is unique, but we know that a sleep cycle takes roughly ninety minutes, so you should be looking to sleep for about 6, 7.5 or 9 hours. Sleep quality trumps sleep quantity every single time, so if you implement the actions in this chapter, you will massively improve your sleep quality, and you may be able to reduce the amount of sleep you need. Finally, I outlined some actions for you to take to help you minimise the impact of jet lag and to help you perform when you land.

Your actions:

∞ Buy a sleep tracking device and track your sleep every night and notice when you have a great night's sleep and when you don't. What did you do the night before?

∞ Complete the exercise to understand how much sleep you need each day, what time you should go to bed and wake up. Experiment with this to find your sweet spot.

∞ Experiment with the strategies in the 'Hacking Sleep' section and discover what works for you.

∞ When you next take a flight, try out the suggestions to beat jet lag and see what works for you.

Part 3 of this book brings all the actions together in an easy-to-follow checklist.

References

1   Von Ruesten, A., Weikert, C., Fietze, I., & Boeing, H. (2012). Association of sleep duration with chronic diseases in the European Prospective Investigation into Cancer and Nutrition (EPIC)-Potsdam study. *PloS one*, 7(1), e30972. PMID: 22295122 – DOI:10.1371/JOURNAL.PONE.0030972

2   Beccuti, G., & Pannain, S. (2011). Sleep and obesity. *Current opinion in clinical nutrition and metabolic care*, 14(4), 402–412. PMID: 21659802 – DOI: 10.1097/MCO.0B013E3283479109

3   Nutt, D., Wilson, S., & Paterson, L. (2008). Sleep disorders as core symptoms of depression. *Dialogues in clinical neuroscience*, 10(3), 329–336. PMID: 18979946 Retrieved from https://pdfs.semanticscholar.org/734e/decb4e4907bdbfd74d1b2ad06299baf17551.pdf

4   Shan, Z., Ma, H., Xie, M., Yan, P., Guo, Y., Bao, W., & Liu, L. (2015). Sleep duration and risk of type 2 diabetes: a meta-analysis of prospective studies. *Diabetes care*, 38(3), 529–537. PMID: 25715415 – DOI: 10.2337/DC14-2073

5   Spurgeon, D. (2002). People who sleep for seven hours a night live longest. *BMJ: British Medical Journal*, 324(7335), 446. PMCID: 1172056 – DOI: 10.1136/BMJ.324.7335.446/E

6   Heatley E., Harris M., Battersby M., McEvoy R., Chai-Coetzer C., & Antic N. (2013). Obstructive sleep apnoea in adults: A common chronic condition in need of a comprehensive chronic condition management approach. *Sleep Medicine Reviews*, 17(5), 349–355. PMID: 23434125 – DOI: 10.1016/J.SMRV.2012.09.004

7   Ferriss, T. (2016, October 13). My Evening Routine for Optimal Relaxation and Sleep. Retrieved from https://tim.blog/2016/10/13/my-evening-routine-for-optimal-relaxation-and-sleep

CHAPTER FIVE

WHAT GETS MEASURED GETS MANAGED

If you don't set a baseline standard for what you'll accept in life, you'll find it's easy to slip into behaviours and attitudes or a quality of life that's far below what you deserve.

TONY ROBBINS

In this chapter you will discover:

∞ Why it's important to set a baseline and track your progress

∞ The core metrics to track

∞ The physical metrics to track and which ones give the best indicators

∞ How to measure how stressed you are

∞ Which blood biomarkers to track

∞ How to get insights from your hormones, DNA and your gut microbiome

Remember to look out for the recommended resources symbol ®.

Why track?

If you want to make a significant change then you need to know where you're currently at, where you want to get to and be able to monitor your progress along the way. Setting a baseline and measuring incremental improvements will help to motivate you and move you forward. There are a wide range of biomarkers to track and it may at first seem overwhelming. Thankfully, the quantified-self movement has exploded over the past few years with the introduction of wearables. Fitness and health trackers give us the ability to measure critical biomarkers at home and some can track multiple biometrics.

Tracking your biomarkers is going to give you further insight into how you are feeling, how you're performing and what your energy levels are like. Given your mitochondria are responsible for most of your energy production then tracking metrics that directly relate to your energy levels is essential.

Core metrics – activity and sleep

Tracking your sleep and activity are the two most essential and popular metrics for you to track. If you track nothing else, make sure you monitor your activity and sleep.

Activity tracking

Activity tracking is one of the most popular metrics to track and has been driven by the infamous need to take 10,000 steps per day. I remember when I was young, arriving home from school one day and my mother had a pedometer to track her steps as part of an office competition.

MYTH: You need to walk 10,000 steps per day.

TRUTH: This is a number that originated from a Japanese marketing campaign which capitalised on the success of the 1964 Tokyo Olympics. The company Yamasa designed the world's first wearable step-counter called a manpo-kei, which translates to '10,000-step meter'. You do need to move frequently, but the intensity of the movement is what matters most.

Fortunately, many of the activity trackers on the market now do a lot more than just track your steps. When selecting a device ® to monitor your activity, make sure it's waterproof and it records all activity including idle time and intensity. I cover more on activity in Chapter 7.

Sleep

Sleep is the cornerstone of your performance and having good quality and duration of sleep is critically important to your performance today and on subsequent days. Tracking your sleep ® is, without a doubt, the most important metric to follow because it will change your behaviour and increase your performance. Sleep is the sole subject of Chapter 4.

There are many sleep devices on the market, and many of them make bold claims but aren't backed up by scientific research and are inaccurate. When selecting a sleep tracking device, look for one that:

- ∞ Has been independently verified

- ∞ Measures not only your quantity of sleep (length) but more importantly the quality of your sleep including your deep sleep, light sleep, rapid eye movement (REM) sleep and when you're awake

∞ Measures your Heart Rate Variability (HRV)

Some sleep devices will also enable you to track your body temperature which will allow you to get insight into if your body is fighting infection or viruses, or, for the ladies, it will show if you're ovulating. One summer, I picked up a nasty insect bite, which became big, red and itchy and that night I had a terrible night's sleep. When I woke up the next morning my sleep device told me that my body temperature was one degree above average, so I knew that my body was fighting an infection.

CASE STUDY: Jim was having difficulty sleeping and was waking up early in the morning and unable to get back to sleep. He started to track his sleep each evening, with a device that measured not only his sleep but also his HRV and body temperature. By simply monitoring his sleep and wanting a good sleep score, his mindset switched to focus on his amount of deep sleep and what was impacting his resting heart rate at night. Jim's sleep improved dramatically as he discovered what he needed to avoid before bedtime.

Physical biometrics

Weight

I weigh myself ® every day to monitor my inflammation and I've done it for many years. If my weight has increased in the past twenty-four hours, then it's usually associated with inflammation because I've eaten or drunk something I shouldn't have. I also find that my weight can spike from one day to the next if I haven't moved enough in the previous day.

Waist-height ratio

This is a straightforward measurement to take, measure your waist (one inch above your belly button) and height in centimetres and divide your waist by your height.

1. > 0.5 – signifies a higher risk of diabetes[1] and heart disease[2]

2. < 0.5 – is considered healthy

MYTH: BMI (Body Mass Index) is a reliable predictor of health.

TRUTH: BMI is a biomarker created in the 1800s by the Belgian mathematician Adolphe Quetelet. Unfortunately, it is still one of the most popular biomarkers that health practitioners use to predict your health, but it's out of date because it doesn't consider how much muscle you are carrying and how much fat is around your middle. Muscular people often have a high BMI score, and people with skinny legs can have a low score. You're better off using the waist to height ratio.

Body fat percentage

It's challenging to measure your actual body fat, and most of the methods give you an estimate. The most popular ways to track body fat are:

- ∞ Calipers – the pinch test and for a small amount of money they are surprisingly accurate ®

- ∞ Weighing scales – these are flawed and inaccurate, so I don't recommend them

- ∞ Dual-energy X-ray absorptiometry (DEXA) scan – is an expensive option but the most accurate ®

The following table provides guidelines on percentage of body fat for women and men:

Description	Women	Men
Essential Fat	10–13%	2–5%
Athletes	14–20%	6–13%
Fitness	21–24%	14–17%
Average	25–31%	18–24%
Obese	32%+	25%+

Blood pressure

High blood pressure is referred to as the 'silent killer' because you can feel fine and then suddenly you could have a heart attack or stroke. Sorry to be so morbid but it's something that's worth keeping a close eye on, even if you don't have a history of high blood pressure. Blood pressure monitors ® are inexpensive, and you can use them at home and synchronise them to your smartphone. When you measure your blood pressure, you have two readings and the following table provides the ranges associated with blood pressure:

	Systolic (top reading)	Diastolic (bottom reading)
Ideal	90–120	60–80
Pre-high blood pressure	120–140	80–90
High blood pressure	Over 140	Over 90

Tracking stress

Many online tests, quizzes and surveys claim to be able to predict your stress levels, but they are inaccurate and take time to complete. The most accurate measure of stress that I've found is to measure your Heart Rate Variability (HRV).

I cover HRV in Chapter 11, so I'm not going to give a detailed explanation in this chapter but tracking your HRV is a critical biomarker that indicates your overall health. Look for a device ® that is convenient; many HRV trackers require you to wear a chest strap ® with the tracker located close to your heart. These are fine if you are looking to track your HRV over a more extended period but are inconvenient if you want a one-off reading.

Blood biomarkers

Getting an understanding of your blood markers will not only save you thousands on supplements but will also focus your attention on improving your overall energy levels. Some doctors do not provide you with these tests unless you're showing specific symptoms, so you may need to purchase these tests privately. It's best to work with a Functional Medical Practitioner to help you analyse your results, and don't worry if any of them are showing in the abnormal range. What is normal for you isn't normal for somebody else.

Basic blood markers

The following blood markers are the basic ⓡ ones that you should be looking to test:

- ∞ Complete blood count – including the number of white and red blood cells.

- ∞ Vitamin D – 50% of my clients have low vitamin D levels, and vitamin D is essential for your energy levels, immune system, metabolism, bone strength and muscle strength.

- ∞ Vitamin B12 – Vitamin B12 is vital for your DNA synthesis, production of blood cells and proper functioning of your nervous system. An Active B12 test is best.

- ∞ Liver and kidney function – your kidneys and liver detoxify your body of harmful pollutants from your everyday environment. Poor liver and kidney health can lead to chronic disease, unwanted weight gain and loss of energy.

- ∞ Haemoglobin A1c (HbA1C) is a marker of your average blood sugar level over the last three months and is an indicator if you are pre-diabetic.

- ∞ High sensitivity C-reactive protein (hs-CRP) is a marker of how much inflammation you have in your body.

∞ Blood lipids – this will include high-density lipoprotein (HDL), low-density lipoprotein (LDL) and triglycerides. The following ratios are good indicators of heart disease:

~ Triglyceride / HDL ratio: It is also a good indicator for predicting your lipoprotein particle size (two or lower is good, and anything over four needs to be addressed).

~ Total cholesterol / HDL ratio – a ratio above five is considered high risk.

MYTH: High LDL cholesterol is always a bad sign.

TRUTH: If you have high LDL cholesterol and you are living a well-balanced lifestyle, then you may not necessarily be high risk for cardiovascular disease. Before you consider taking statins, ask your doctor to check for the following:

∞ ApoB (Apolipoprotein B) – helps bind LDL cholesterol and therefore clog blood vessels. ApoB is a good indicator of cardiovascular risk.

∞ Lipid particle numbers and sizes – large fluffy LDL particles act as protective cholesterol in the same way as HDL cholesterol, whereas the small dense LDL particles cross into your arteries and harden them.

∞ High sensitivity C-reactive protein (hs-CRP) – as discussed earlier, this is a measure of inflammation in the body.

Advanced blood markers

The following blood markers ® are more specialised and are extremely useful:

∞ Insulin-like growth factor-1 (IGF-1) – needs to be balanced to promote healthy cells. However, high IGF-1 and cancer could promote cancerous growth.

∞ Advanced cholesterol – Many blood tests will provide you with your HDL and LDL cholesterol levels. This isn't enough information; you want to look for a test that provides you with more detail around the LDL proteins, particle numbers and sizes.

∞ Homocysteine – is linked with cardiovascular disease and Alzheimer's disease.

∞ Ferritin – is a measure of your iron levels.

∞ Magnesium – is of critical importance in the body and is responsible for many bodily functions. Most people are deficient in magnesium because it's increasingly difficult to get it from food.[3]

∞ Omega-6 content of the mitochondrial membranes – healthy mitochondria need the right proportions of omega-6 and omega-3 fatty acids. The ideal ratio is 4:1. Too much omega-6 can make the mitochondria prone to oxidative stress.[4]

Hormone panel

Your body uses hormones for a variety of critical bodily functions, and they are a great indicator of how healthy you are.

Hormones are used to build tissue, babies, and help you to lead a robust life. They will decrease and change over time, but you shouldn't just accept low hormone levels. There is usually an underlying cause and adjusting your hormone levels could make a big difference to your energy and performance.

The best hormone tests ® are those where you can take urine samples multiple times per day with information on your metabolites, which is the underlying pathology behind each hormone.

Gut microbiome testing

Microbiome testing ® is proving to be one of the most exciting developments.

All disease begins in the gut.

Hippocrates

This quote from Hippocrates has stood the test of time and originated around 2,000 years ago. It's a strong statement to make and one that has a lot of merit and credibility as a result of recent scientific discoveries. It's not 100% accurate because there are genetic diseases, but scientists are now looking into an imbalanced gut microbiome as the source of many chronic diseases.

All over your body, around your skin and from your mouth down to your colon, you have a collection of microbes, referred to as the microbiome. Apart from your skin, your gut contains the highest concentration of microbes on your body, referred to as the gut microbiome, and it is a complex mix of bacteria, fungi, viruses and archaea.

When you eat, you're not just eating for energy for yourself, but you're also eating for the trillions of microbes in your gut, which are responsible for producing vitamins and hormones.

Your gut microbiome plays a critical role in communicating with your immune system to tell it which of the microbes are pathogens, so they are kept out of your body. Your gut microbiome is also responsible for producing many of the nutrients that your mitochondria need to perform optimally.

Many diseases start in the gut,[5] so looking after your gut microbiome is essential. These tests are not exactly glamorous because you need to provide a stool sample, but hey, it's only your poo.

DNA testing

DNA testing is popular because it enables you to track your ancestry and discover what you may be pre-disposed to. For example, you may discover how likely you are to go bald, how well you process caffeine and risk factors associated with chronic disease.

There are two essential elements to consider:

1. Taking your DNA – the key thing here is to ensure that the service you use enables you to export your DNA for loading into other services ®

2. Analysing your DNA – look for a trusted site that has a solid privacy policy and is clear on how accurate their results are ®

There is an important point to understand when it comes to DNA testing. If you find genetic information that points towards a concerning condition, it does not mean that that condition is going to occur. It's how your genes express themselves through epigenetics that matters most, and your environment dictates this. Therefore, focus on your symptoms and use your DNA results to help you understand the root cause but please don't run off and start trying to treat something that may not exist.

Summary

Creating a baseline and tracking against it is a great way to make progress and see the results. If you do nothing else, track the basics, which is your sleep and activity levels. Tracking additional physical biometrics is also useful and includes your weight, height to waist ratio, body fat and blood pressure. Stress is a massive issue for executives and entrepreneurs so measuring your Heart Rate Variability is essential, so you can track your stress levels and recovery time. Your blood markers and hormone levels provide insightful information on what is going on in your body and therefore how you are feeling and performing. Finally, more advanced metrics to track that give great insights are your DNA and gut microbiome.

Your actions:

∞ Measure and track your activity and the quality of your sleep each night ®

∞ Track your physical biomarkers and set a reminder to review them on a regular basis

∞ Measure your Heart Rate Variability to track your stress and recovery levels ®

- ∞ Purchase a basic blood panel ® or ask your doctor for the tests

- ∞ If you wish to go deeper, purchase a more advanced blood panel ® and a hormone panel ®

- ∞ Purchase a DNA test ® and run the results through online diagnostic tools ®

- ∞ Have your gut microbiome tested ®

Part 3 of this book brings all the actions together in an easy-to-follow checklist.

References

1   Jamar, G., Almeida, F., Gagliardi, A., Sobral, M., Ping, C., Sperandio, E., Romiti, M., Arantes R., & Dourado, V. (2017). Evaluation of waist-to-height ratio as a predictor of insulin resistance in non-diabetic obese individuals. A cross-sectional study. *Sao Paulo Medical Journal*, 135(5), 462–468. PMID: 29116305 – DOI: 10.1590/1516-3180.2016.0358280417

2   Rådholm, K., Chalmers, J., Ohkuma, T., Peters, S., Poulter, N., Hamet, P., Harrap, S., & Woodward M. (2018). Use of the waist-to-height ratio to predict cardiovascular risk in patients with diabetes: Results from the ADVANCE-ON study. *Diabetes, obesity and metabolism,* 20(8), 1903–1910. PMID: 29603537 – DOI: 10.1111/DOM.13311

3   DiNicolantonio, J. J., O'Keefe, J. H., & Wilson, W. (2018). Subclinical magnesium deficiency: a principal driver of cardiovascular disease and a public health crisis. *Open heart*, 5(1), e000668. PMID: 29387426 – DOI: 10.1136/OPENHRT-2017-000668

4   Patterson, E., Wall, R., Fitzgerald, G. F., Ross, R. P., & Stanton, C. (2012). Health implications of high dietary omega-6 polyunsaturated Fatty acids. *Journal of nutrition and metabolism*, 2012, 539426. PMID: 22570770 – DOI: 10.1155/2012/539426

5   Bull, M. J., & Plummer, N. T. (2014). Part 1: The Human Gut Microbiome in Health and Disease. *Integrative medicine (Encinitas, Calif.)*, 13(6), 17–22. PMID: 26770121

CHAPTER SIX

BURNING FAT FOR FUEL

I fast for greater physical and mental efficiency.

PLATO

In this chapter you will discover:

- ∞ The sources of energy and macronutrients; and why fat isn't bad

- ∞ How fasting creates ketones which boost your performance and helps your body cleanse itself through a process called autophagy

- ∞ How to build fasting into your life with intermittent fasting

- ∞ The benefits of one-day and three-day water-only fasts

Remember to look out for the recommended resources symbol **Ⓡ**.

Fat is back

Nutrients are what feed your cells, and they fall into two types, essential nutrients and non-essential nutrients:

1. Non-essential nutrients are crucial, so don't let the name confuse you. It just means that your body can

make these nutrients. For example, vitamin D, some amino acids and cholesterol.

2. Essential nutrients are those that must be derived from your diet and so your body cannot make them. These include:

   i.   Macronutrients – fats, protein and carbohydrates

   ii. Micronutrients – some vitamins, minerals and water

For energy, your body can burn carbohydrates (glucose), protein or fats (fatty acids), and while protein can also be metabolised into energy, it's not an efficient process. It is also critical to maintain metabolic flexibility, so your body needs to be able to switch between burning fatty acids and burning glucose.

Fat, particularly saturated fat, had a bad reputation during the 1980s and 1990s as the sugar industry proliferated. Sugar then became bad, and the artificial sweetener craze started. The low-fat craze has gone too far, but slowly the balance is being redressed.

The following is a breakdown of the different types of fats:

∞ Monounsaturated – avocados, olives, olive oil, cashews, hazelnuts

∞ Polyunsaturated – oily fish, flaxseeds, sunflower seeds, walnuts

∞ Saturated – meat, butter, ghee and coconut oil

∞ Trans – fried foods, snacks, cakes, pastries, takeaways. Avoid these fats at all costs because nobody should be eating these foods, they are toxic and the World Health

Organization has called on all governments to remove them from food supplies by 2023.[1] There are no known benefits to eating trans-fat. You may also hear of transfats under the label of hydrogenated oils or PHOs

The stability of the fats is critical, especially when they are cooked or start to spoil because they become inflammatory. The most stable to unstable fats are: saturated, monounsaturated and then polyunsaturated.

It's for this reason that you should never cook on high heat with oils such as sunflower oil or olive oil because they oxidise at low temperatures. It would be best if you cooked with butter, ghee or coconut oil.

MYTH: Saturated fat is bad for you.

TRUTH: Saturated fat consumption was once linked to cardiovascular disease, so the public health advice was to minimise saturated fat and therefore eggs, butter and red meat were demonised. This is still the advice given today by the American Heart Association despite a 2010 review[2] which performed a meta-analysis of 347,747 subjects and concluded that:

'A meta-analysis of prospective epidemiologic studies showed that there is no significant evidence for concluding that dietary saturated fat is associated with an increased risk of coronary heart disease or coronary vascular disease.'

Another review in 2014[3] of over 600,000 participants and funded by the British Heart Foundation concluded that:

'Current evidence does not clearly support cardiovascular guidelines that encourage high consumption of polyunsaturated fatty acids and low consumption of total saturated fats.'

Two of the most important types of fat are found in polyun-saturated fats and are called omega-3s (O3s) and omega-6s (O6s). You can only get these fats from your diet and O3s are anti-inflammatory while O6s are inflammatory, so you need to maximise the O3s and minimise the O6s. O3s include three different types of fatty acids, EPA (eicosapentaenoic acid), DHA (docosahexaenoic acid) and ALA (alpha-linolenic acid).

An ideal ratio is no more than 4:1 (06 to 03). However, it estimated that in developed countries, the ratio is closer to 16:1.

In *Resources,* I've provided a list of foods ⓡ with their O6/ O3 ratios, some notable ones are covered in the following table:

	O6 (grams)	O3 (grams)	Ratio
Salmon	0.2	2.3	1 to 12
Sardines	4	1.8	2.2 to 1
Mackerel	0.2	2.2	1 to 11
Cashew Nuts	2.179	0.017	125 to 1
Flax Seeds	1.655	6.388	1 to 4
Pumpkin Seeds	2.452	0.021	114 to 1

Ketosis

When you go without food and fast and the liver has used up its supply of glycogen (carbohydrates) the body switches to its fat stores to produce energy. This is a metabolic state called ketosis where your body is using fat as its primary energy source and is producing ketone bodies, which fuel your mitochondria. When your mitochondria use ketones rather than glucose as a fuel source they're able to generate more energy per unit of oxygen. Ketosis can also be simulated through dietary sources such as medium-chain triglyceride (MCT) oil ®.

When you're in ketosis, you feel like you're in a state of high performance, and you have a surge of calm energy with crystal clear mental clarity. You're burning fat, and you don't feel hungry.

Ketosis not only burns fat but it also:

- ∞ Prevents you from being hungry by regulating your hunger hormones, leptin and ghrelin.

- ∞ Increases neurotransmitter levels gamma-aminobutyric acid (GABA), up-regulates your mitochondrial energy and increases your brain power. Remember that you have ten times more mitochondria in your brain.

Most people now live on a carbohydrate-heavy diet which tells your body that there is a plentiful supply of energy and there is no need for it to go into your fat stores to burn fat. If we go back a couple of thousand years, there wasn't the abundance of grains that we have now, and our diet was very much feast and fast. We would rely on being in a ketogenic state to survive between meals. These days, few people get to experience a state of ketosis.

Cutting your carbohydrate load isn't enough to put you into a state of ketosis, you also need to cut down on your protein because your body will convert the protein you eat to energy. To put yourself into a state of ketosis, you need to fast for a period; usually, for at least fourteen hours. This depletes your body of glycogen, and your body then turns to its fat stores. It can take a while for your body to become fat adapted, so you may find that you get hungry in the first few days.

It's possible to measure your level of ketosis using either ketone urine strips ⊙ or a blood ketone monitor ⊙. I have found that the urine strips are not accurate enough and only provide a rough approximation, whereas the blood ketone meter can detect the level of ketones in your blood beta-hydroxybutyrate (BHB).

When using the blood meter, the following measurements will tell you the level of ketosis that you're achieving:

Reading (mmol/L)	Ketogenic state
0.2–0.5	Mild ketosis
0.5	Nutritional ketosis, where your hunger hormones ghrelin and leptin are regulated
1.5–3.0	Optimal ketosis for fat-burning and where you experience the effects of mental clarity
10 +	Ketoacidosis: This is a life-threatening condition usually associated with untreated diabetes and alcoholism, and you can't hit this level by a ketogenic diet alone

Why fasting is good for you

Fasting has been a way of life during many religious festivals for thousands of years and not because resources were scarce. As part of Yom Kippur, Jews will abstain from food and drink and ask for forgiveness. For the month of Ramadan, Muslims abstain from food and liquids during the day and break the fast with a meal after sundown.

What do they know that we don't?

Fasting has some incredible benefits, and the most significant benefit is promoting a process called autophagy. Autophagy is a Greek word which means to eat oneself and is a metabolic process that enables your body to cleanse itself naturally. The understanding of this mechanism has increased in the past few years, and in 2016 the Nobel Prize in Physiology or Medicine was awarded to Yoshinori Ohsumi for *'his discoveries of mechanisms for autophagy – a fundamental process for degrading and recycling cellular components.'*

Autophagy is the body's system of cleaning out and recycling parts of dead, diseased or worn-out cells. Your body can clean out the inside of the cells and use the resulting molecules for energy or to make new parts of cells. In Part One of this book, you learned about apoptosis, which is programmed cell death, but autophagy is different because it enables sub-cellular regeneration.

Many chronic diseases such as cancer, Alzheimer's and Parkinson's are linked to excess defective and abnormal proteins and organelles in the cells. Autophagy removes this debris, so your cells can function optimally.

Ancient religions knew this was good for them even though the science at the time didn't support it. Autophagy is unique to fasting, and you cannot achieve it through dieting or restricting calories.

MYTH:	**Breakfast is the most important meal of the day.**
TRUTH:	How many times have you heard your parents say this to you when you were younger? When you are asleep, you are in a fasted state, and often when you wake up, you are thirsty rather than hungry. Try having a large glass of water. Much of what people eat in the morning is not good for them because it's high in carbohydrates which spikes your insulin levels and causes a crash later in the morning. If you feel hungry in the morning, then it's best to have something protein-based.

Intermittent fasting

There have been many forms of fasting diets over the past few years, and perhaps one of the most popular has been the 5:2 diet, which is a form of intermittent fasting and involves eating a reduced number of calories (typically 600) for two consecutive days each week.

Many people find this form of intermittent fasting to be tough going, and they only get the benefits of fasting for two days per week. A better form of intermittent fasting is to eat within a six-hour window between the hours of 2pm and 8pm and fast for eighteen hours each day.

Intermittent fasting in this way enables you to eat two meals per day and the timing can be flexible based on what you're doing that day, but always aim to fast between sixteen to eighteen hours per day. It does take a little bit of practice, and I'd recommend you start with a shorter fasting window, say fourteen hours, and build it up slowly. You may struggle for the first few days as your body becomes fat adapted so don't rush it, take it slowly.

When you are fasting, you need to limit the number of carbohydrates to thirty to fifty grams per day. This way it keeps your glycogen levels low enough to quickly deplete so that your body enters ketosis. Carbohydrates are an important macronutrient, so I recommend that you cycle in and out of ketosis so that you maintain metabolic flexibility. Therefore, only fast for five or six days per week.

Bulletproof® Coffee got me started with biohacking and was the first thing I've found that turned on my brain and made me feel highly energised. I have consistently had a cup every morning for the past two years, and I'll go well out of my way to find or make one. To make Bulletproof® Coffee, you blend:

1. A cup of Bulletproof® Coffee ®

2. One tablespoon of grass-fed butter ®

3. One tablespoon of Bulletproof® Brain Octane® ®

The next step is to blend all the ingredients for at least thirty seconds, and the result is a coffee that is very much like a latte. Trust me. It's not disgusting; it's delicious. The advantages of a Bulletproof® Coffee are:

∞ It helps to regulates your hunger hormones

∞ The Brain Octane® oil contains exogenous ketones which your brain loves using for energy. I mentioned dietary sources of exogenous ketones earlier in this chapter

∞ The butter and caffeine combination slowly releases the caffeine, rather than the usual spike and crash

∞ It provides enough energy to sustain you through your intermittent fast

Twenty-four-hour water fasting

A water fast is where the only thing you consume for that period is water, so no food or other liquids. This has the benefits of pushing your body deeper into a state of ketosis, and you can reap significant benefits from autophagy. I perform a twenty-four hour fast whenever I need to skip a meal, and this may be because I'm at an event and there is no suitable food or if I'm on an aeroplane. A twenty-four hour fast may feel like a step too far right now, but it's a lot easier than you think, especially once you have been intermittent fasting for some time.

Three-day water fasting

Experimenting with a twenty-four hour fast is unlikely to do you any harm, but with a three-day water fast, there is more risk because you could become weak and pass out. Please do your research and consult a Functional Medical Practitioner if you have any underlying medical conditions. Never conduct a three-day water fast unless you are comfortable doing a twenty-four hour fast.

A three-day fast is going to put you deep into ketosis and maximise the benefits from autophagy.

- ∞ Day one of the fast is uneventful and easy because it's a standard twenty-four hour fast

- ∞ Day two is tough, energy levels start to dip, and it can be a struggle at times but it's worth it

- ∞ Day three is euphoric, you have a burst of good clean energy, and your cognition is superb

When you break your fast, do it slowly, don't binge eat and consume the foods you would typically eat.

> **CASE STUDY:** Tim had been intermittent fasting for some time and tried a few twenty-four-hour fasts. He wanted to go deeper and try a five-day water fast. I suggested that he try a three-day water fast first and maybe next time try a five-day water fast. When I saw him for his coaching session, he was on day five already and said that he had never felt better in his life. He described the benefits that he had experienced as: mental clearness, clarity of thought processes, weight stability and detoxing not only his body but also his mind.

Summary

Your body needs carbohydrates, fat and protein to survive and consuming the right types of fat is critically important to your energy levels. Saturated fat isn't the 'bad fat' and you should focus on eating foods with a ratio of Omega 6s to Omega 3s as close to 4 to 1 as you can.

Most people are living a carbohydrate-rich lifestyle, and their bodies don't have the metabolic flexibility to be able to switch between burning fat and burning carbohydrates. By lowering your carbohydrate intake, increasing your healthy fat consumption and eating between the hours of 2pm and 8pm, you can enter a metabolic state called ketosis that not only makes you feel highly energised but also induces autophagy, which is your body's natural ability to clean up at a cellular level.

Your actions:

∞ Check out the *Resources* and identify the foods higher in Omega 3s and build them into your diet ®

∞ Try a cup of Bulletproof® Coffee ® in the morning and see how you feel when the exogenous ketones hit your brain

∞ Cut back your carbohydrates to 30–50g a day

∞ Measure your ketones using a ketone blood monitor ®

∞ Eat two meals a day between the hours of 2pm and 8pm. If you find it difficult, build it up slowly

∞ Try a twenty-four-hour fast one day when there is nothing suitable to eat

∞ Step up to a three-day fast to experience the benefits of being deep in ketosis

Part 3 of this book brings all the actions together in an easy-to-follow checklist.

References

1   Thornton, J. (2018). Eliminate "toxic" trans fats from food by 2023, WHO urges. Retrieved from www.bmj.com/content/361/bmj.k2154

2   Siri-Tarino, P. W., Sun, Q., Hu, F. B., & Krauss, R. M. (2010). Meta-analysis of prospective cohort studies evaluating the association of saturated fat with cardiovascular disease. *The American journal of clinical nutrition*, 91(3), 535–546. PMID: 20071648 – DOI: 10.3945/AJCN.2009.27725

3   Chowdhury, R., Warnakula, S., Kunutsor, S., Crowe, F., Ward, H. A., Johnson, L., ... & Khaw, K. T. (2014). Association of dietary, circulating, and supplement fatty acids with coronary risk: a systematic review and meta-analysis. *Annals of internal medicine*, 160(6), 398–406. PMID: 24723079 – DOI: 10.7326/M13-1788

CHAPTER SEVEN

MOVE MORE AND EXERCISE LESS

The bottom line is that a single set taken to the point of positive failure is a sufficient stimulus to trigger the growth and strength mechanism of the body into motion. Additional sets produce nothing but more time spent in the gym.

DR DOUG MCGUFF
AUTHOR OF *BODY BY SCIENCE*

In this chapter you will discover:

- ∞ Why over-exercising isn't the best strategy

- ∞ How High-Intensity Interval Training maximises your return on investment

- ∞ Why movement is as important as exercise

- ∞ How to experience grounding

Remember to look out for the recommended resources symbol ®.

Don't over-exercise

This chapter is going to be particularly contentious for people who love doing endurance exercise. If you are running or cycling long distances in the pursuit of being healthy you aren't doing any favours for your health and performance.

I meet many senior leaders and entrepreneurs who complain about having a demanding job and that they don't get to see enough of their family, yet they find the time to train for an ultra-marathon, go on three-hour bike rides or spend hours in the gym each week. They do this because they feel that they are putting themselves and their health first.

I'm not judging, because it is always a challenge to strike the right balance between health, family time and work. As I covered earlier in the book, most people put health at the bottom of their list of priorities; but those people who dedicate so much time to exercise, unfortunately, aren't doing as much to promote their health and performance as they think. The problem is that they are exposed to stress, and the combination of a demanding job, busy family life and over-exercising is a dangerous mix because exercise causes more stress on the body.

In general, many people are resting too much, have too much desk time and are inactive. On the other side, people who are interested in exercise often destroy the balance by going to the other extreme and don't focus enough on recovery.

Exercise is a form of stress, and it momentarily weakens you to get an adaptive response that makes you stronger. Busy people are continually experiencing chronic amounts of stress and exercise adds to it. Stress results from many sources including:

- ∞ Poor sleep quality and quantity

- ∞ Toxic relationships

- ∞ Work pressures

Many people have been pre-programmed to think that being very slim and hugely active is the elixir of being healthy. However, it couldn't be further from the truth. It's not how you look on the outside that determines your health, but it's what's going on inside your body that matters. A 2017 study[1] evaluated 2,175 participants over a twenty-five-year period and found that white males who exercised three times the weekly average were at higher odds of developing hardening of the arteries by their middle age.

MYTH: **To get a six pack you need to hit the gym.**

TRUTH: If you want a great six pack for the beach, then stop focusing so much on the gym and concentrate on what you put on your plate. Great abs come from what you put on your plate and not what you do in the gym. You can work out for hours in the gym, but if you are consuming too many carbohydrates, then you are going to struggle to drop your body fat percentage to be able to see your abdominal muscles.

I'm not criticising people who spend hours exercising; if it works for you, then that's great. However, there is another way to achieve a high level of health and fitness, and that's by making sure you move every day and perform high-intensity exercise three times a week.

High-intensity interval training

The popularity of High-Intensity Interval Training (HIIT) has grown in recent years, and as such there are many apps which provide guided instructions on how to perform HIIT. The great thing with HIIT is that you regain so much time and your exercise routine can fit around you regardless of vacation days, whether you are at home or travelling away on business.

The most accessible form of HIIT is the seven-minute workout Ⓡ, where you perform nine exercises for forty seconds each with a ten second break between them. There are slight variations on the exercises depending on the app you select, but the most common sequence is:

1. Jumping jacks

2. Wall seat

3. Lunge

4. Press-up

5. Sit up

6. Triceps dips

7. Plank

8. Rotation press-ups

9. High knees

In just seven minutes your heart will be pumping, and you'll be sweating a lot. This is a great way to get started with an exercise practice if you don't have one, and if you are already fit and active, you can repeat the seven-minute workout two or three times to give yourself a fourteen-minute workout or twenty-one-minute workout. By taking seven, fourteen or twenty-one minutes two or three times a week, you will see your body shape change significantly, and you will lose weight.

> **EXERCISE: Try a fast HIIT workout.**
>
> Go to your favourite App Store and type in *'7-minute workout'* and download one of the many free apps. Take some time today or tomorrow to try out HIIT for just seven minutes.

There are many other ways to perform HIIT:

1. Sprint for thirty seconds as fast as you possibly can, lie on your back for thirty seconds, get back up and sprint again for thirty seconds and repeat this cycle six times.

2. Use a cross-trainer and go hard for sixty seconds followed by sixty seconds at a moderate pace and repeat ten times.

3. Row for four minutes, rest for one minute and repeat four times.

4. Sprint, push-ups and squats – sprint for fifteen seconds, then ten push-ups and followed by ten squats. Rest for thirty seconds and then repeat. This will hit all of the key areas of your body. Do as many rounds as you can.

There are many studies that prove that HIIT exercise for a short amount of time has the same benefits of a much longer workout. Here are just a few examples:

∞ Sports scientists at Canada's McMaster University found that just three twenty-second sprints at maximum effort followed by two minutes of medium-intensity provides the same improvement to your cardiorespiratory system as forty-five minutes of medium-intensity exercise.[2]

∞ A study published by the American Journal of Cardiovascular Disease compared the results on HIIT and moderate intensity training for women at risk of hypertension. After sixteen weeks the HITT group showed the most significant improvements to blood pressure and insulin sensitivity.[3]

∞ The American Council on Exercise conducted a study to evaluate the effectiveness of HIIT resistance training. It found that HIIT resistance training is as effective as traditional time-intensive weightlifting programmes.[4]

During HIIT your heart rate will increase, so you need to know how high you can safely go. Your maximum heart rate drops with age, and a good rule of thumb is to subtract your age from 220. I'm 41, so my maximum heart rate is 179. This maximum can change depending on any medications that you are taking or your general health. When performing HIIT you want to take your heart rate to 80–90% of its maximum, so for me, it would be 144–161 beats per minute.

Strength training

HIIT isn't just limited to cardio-based exercise and is equally applicable to strength training. In 1964, Arthur Jones pioneered the thinking behind High-Intensity Strength Training and founded his own set of exercise equipment called Nautilus. Dr Doug McGuff, the author of *Body by Science,* has written extensively on this subject, and his strength training programme can be completed in just twelve minutes, once per week.

When you perform HIIT strength training, you work your muscles to rapid fatigue, and in doing so, you can increase muscle faster and in the fraction of the time of conventional strength training.

CASE STUDY: When I attended the Bulletproof® Conference in Pasadena in October 2017, I was eager to check out the guys from ARX ®, who were exhibiting at the conference. ARX stands for adaptive resistance exercise and is computer-controlled exercise equipment, which enables you to have a full body workout in twenty minutes, and you only need to perform it once a week. I tried out a single exercise on the ARX, the leg press. I settled into the seat and slowly pushed out the pad with my legs; the ARX then slowly moves back towards you, and you must resist on the backward motion. The ARX matches your strength perfectly, so as you get weaker, it lowers the resistance. This means that it can be used by the super strong or the elderly. The workout was immense, and after only two minutes, I could feel that my legs were fatigued.

This is just one example of how strength training is being revolutionised. As I'm writing this book, I'm experimenting with a piece of strength training equipment that can be used at home; it doesn't take up much space and promises to build muscle three times faster ⑬.

Strength training is perceived to be all about building muscle mass and having a great body for the beach, but it's much more important than superficial cosmetics. Strength training has been shown to:

∞ Increase bone density.[5] Strong bones are vital to overall health and help avoid osteoporosis and fractures.

∞ A 2010 review[6] summarised the findings from several randomised controlled studies and found that strength training improves anxiety, cognition, sleep quality and self-esteem. It also reduces pain associated with the lower back, osteoarthritis and fibromyalgia.

∞ A 2015 study[7] published by Harvard researchers followed 10,500 men over twelve years and found that strength training was more effective at preventing abdominal fat than cardiovascular exercise.

The time savings from HIIT are impressive and it is remarkably beneficial for your energy and mitochondria. A study[8] published in Cell Metabolism found that HIIT improved mitochondrial capacity in younger volunteers by 49% and older volunteers by 69%.

Get moving

Moving is fundamental to your performance, and so many people spend countless hours sitting down, whether it be commuting to work, working at a desk or in front of the TV.

The magical metric associated with movement is 10,000 steps, which originated from Japan and is linked to the pedometer craze in the 1990s. Depending on your occupation, 10,000 steps can be difficult to achieve every day, especially for those who must sit at a desk.

The more that you can move the better, because it's the only way that your lymphatic system shifts lymph around your body to remove waste.

Some easy ways to move more during the day are:

∞ Alternate from sitting to standing and don't sit for longer than fifty minutes

∞ Take the stairs whenever possible

∞ Get off your train or bus a stop earlier on your commute to the office

∞ Use a standing desk Ⓡ and switch between standing and sitting. Standing for long periods of time at a desk is like sitting.

I use a neat hack to cheat my way to 10,000 steps a day by using a vibration plate Ⓡ. I use the plate for five to fifteen minutes each day to help move my lymphatic system and increase my muscle tone. Vibration plates were invented by the Russians as part of their space programme and were used to ensure that while on space missions the astronauts didn't lose muscle tone.

When using the vibration plate, you can stand still, perform exercises such as the plank, stomach crunches and squats, or do yoga.

Not all vibration plates are equal, some are cheap, and others can cost thousands. If you are considering buying one, then look for one that:

∞ Has a large enough base for you to be able to exercise on.

∞ Has an adjustable frequency from 10 to 50Hz. Historically, 30Hz has been the most used frequency, but emerging research is suggesting that 50Hz may have additional benefits.

∞ Only moves vertically and not horizontally. Many cheap vibration plates move vertically and horizontally in a wobble like movement which is bad news for your knee joints.

If you don't have the space for a vibration plate, then a small indoor trampoline works well.

Grounding

If you can get outside and move without your shoes on, then please do take the chance. There is something magical that happens when you get connected to the earth, whether it be your bare feet in the sand or on grass.

Have you ever experienced an instance when you've spent a significant amount of time outdoors in your bare feet, and you've felt an energised state like you're more connected to the earth? It's also a feeling that many people experience while gardening. There is no doubt that being outside in the fresh air and sunlight plays a significant part in this feeling, but so does grounding.

The Earth is negatively charged and your body over time builds up a positive charge. When you connect with the earth through a conductive surface, the negative charge from the Earth enters your body and neutralises the positive charge.

A study conducted in 2015[9] which included the University of California and the University of Oregon concluded that grounding needs the serious attention of clinicians and researchers because it could be a simple and natural strategy to decrease chronic inflammation.

What have you got to lose by going barefoot in your garden or local park? I can't see any downsides.

Summary

Exercise is the key to your emotional, physical and mental health. Not enough exercise is bad for you, but over-exercising is terrible because it's building up stress in your body and will wear out your joints. Time is precious and adopting HIIT into your exercise regime will provide excellent results in a fraction of the time, power up your mitochondria and enable you to spend time doing the things you want to do. By adopting HIIT and moving more, you will be meeting your biological needs for exercise and if you can do it outside, in the sun and with bare feet, then even better.

Your actions:

∞ Consider how much you are exercising. Are you exercising enough or are you over-exercising? What do you need to change?

∞ Bring HIIT into your exercise regime, both cardio and strength based

∞ Move more, find ways to increase the amount of movement you do each day

∞ Use a vibration plate at home or at your local gym

∞ Get outside in your bare feet and connect with the earth

Part 3 of this book brings all the actions together in an easy-to-follow checklist.

References

1   Laddu, D. R., Rana, J. S., Murillo, R., Sorel, M. E., Quesenberry Jr, C. P., Allen, N. B., ... & Lloyd-Jones, D. (2017, November). 25-Year Physical Activity Trajectories and Development of Subclinical Coronary Artery Disease as Measured by Coronary Artery Calcium: The Coronary Artery Risk Development in Young Adults (CARDIA) Study. *Mayo Clinic Proceedings*, 92(11), 1660–1670. PMID: 29050797 – DOI: 10.1016/J.MAYOCP.2017.07.016

2   Gillen, J. B., Martin, B. J., MacInnis, M. J., Skelly, L. E., Tarnopolsky, M. A., & Gibala, M. J. (2016). Twelve weeks of sprint interval training improves indices of cardiometabolic health similar to traditional endurance training despite a five-fold lower exercise volume and time commitment. *PloS one*, 11(4), e0154075. PMID: 27115137 – DOI: 10.1371/JOURNAL.PONE.0154075

3   Ciolac, E. G. (2012). High-intensity interval training and hypertension: maximizing the benefits of exercise? *American journal of cardiovascular disease*, 2(2), 102–10. PMID: 22720199 Retrieved from: https://pdfs.semanticscholar.org/f82c/dccdc42ef760eb5f99300aa2298b19f87f7a.pdf

4   Dalleck, L. C., Smith, F. E., Green, J. D. (2018). Aerobics Instructor Manual: Is HIIT Resistance Exercise Superior to Traditional Resistance Training? A Randomized, Controlled Trial. *American Council on Exercise*. Retrieved from https://acefitnessmediastorage.blob.core.windows.net/webcontent/June2018/ACE_HIITresistanceStudy.pdf

5   Layne, J. E., & Nelson, M. E. (1999). The effects of progressive resistance training on bone density: a review. *Medicine & Science in Sports & Exercise*, 31(1). PMID: 9927006. Retrieved from https://journals.lww.com/acsm-msse/Fulltext/1999/01000/The_effects_of_progressive_resistance_training_on.6.aspx

6   O'Connor, P. J., Herring, M. P., & Caravalho, A. (2010). Mental health benefits of strength training in adults. *American Journal of Lifestyle Medicine*, 4(5), 377–396. DOI: 10.1177/1559827610368771

7   Mekary, R. A., Grøntved, A., Despres, J. P., De Moura, L. P., Asgarzadeh, M., Willett, W. C., ... & Hu, F. B. (2015). Weight training, aerobic physical activities, and long-term waist circumference change in men. *Obesity*, 23(2), 461–467. PMID: 25530447 – DOI: 10.1002/OBY.20949

8   Robinson, M. M., Dasari, S., Konopka, A. R., Johnson, M. L., Manjunatha, S., Esponda, R. R., Carter, R. E., Lanza, I. R., ... Nair, K. S. (2017). Enhanced Protein Translation Underlies Improved Metabolic and Physical Adaptations to Different Exercise Training Modes in Young and Old Humans. *Cell metabolism*, 25(3), 581–592. PMID: 28273480 – DOI: 10.1016/J.CMET.2017.02.009

9   Oschman, J. L., Chevalier, G., & Brown, R. (2015). The effects of grounding (earthing) on inflammation, the immune response, wound healing, and prevention and treatment of chronic inflammatory and autoimmune diseases. *Journal of Inflammation Research*, 8, 83–96. PMID: 25848315 – DOI: 10.2147/JIR.S69656

CHAPTER EIGHT

EMBRACING THE MAGIC OF LIGHT

It is the unqualified result of all my experience with the sick, that second only to their need of fresh air is their need of light, and that it is not only light, but direct sunlight they want.

FLORENCE NIGHTINGALE

In this chapter you will discover:

- ∞ What sunshine comprises and why it's so important to you

- ∞ What is junk light and why you need to avoid it

- ∞ What Irlen Syndrome is and why you should consider being tested

- ∞ If ultraviolet light is bad for you

- ∞ The healing powers of infrared light

- ∞ How to optimise light throughout your day

Remember to look out for the recommended resources symbol **®**.

The wonders of light

Light is something that you probably take for granted; it's just there. The sun rises in the morning, sets in the evening and when you don't have the sun, you have electricity to provide light. Light is information to your body and is critically important to regulate your circadian rhythms, which is your daily biological clock that controls the release of hormones throughout the day. For example, in the morning you will release cortisol, and in the evening, you will release melatonin. Your body is designed to take light from the sun and you can use this information to optimise yourself.

The sun provides you with the full spectrum of light that you need to live a healthy life, and this includes:

- ∞ Ultraviolet light – with a wavelength between 10 to 400 nanometres, it is responsible for your summer tan and vitamin D production. Ultraviolet light is split into UV-A, UV-B and UV-C light.

- ∞ Visible light – with a wavelength between 400 nanometres to 700 nanometres, it provides you with your primary source of light.

- ∞ Infrared light – with a wavelength between 700 nanometres and 1 millimetre, it provides energy and warmth. Infrared light is split into near-infrared (IR-A), mid-infrared (IR-B) and far-infrared (IR-C).

Sunlight is so important, and it's the reason why you will feel happy and full of joy when you're sat in the park, and the sun is bathing your face, or you go for a walk and feel the warmth on your back. It's not just the warmth that the sun gives you but it's also triggering a series of chemical and biological processes that release your feel-good hormone, serotonin. A lack of sunshine has been linked with low levels of serotonin production in the brain which contributes to Seasonal Affective Disorder (SAD).[1]

In addition to triggering hormone release, the sun sends a biological signal to your body to produce vitamin D sulfate. You can supplement with vitamin D, but only sunlight can produce vitamin D sulfate. If you are supplementing with vitamin D, then you need to be careful because you can build up toxic levels in your body. It's for this reason that I only supplement vitamin D during the winter months. When your body produces vitamin D from sunlight and reaches the optimal level, it stops production.

Light acts like a drug. There, I said it.

Am I crazy?

I don't think so.

There are many benefits associated with having sun exposure and they include:

∞ Improvement of skin conditions such as eczema,[2] jaundice[3] and psoriasis.[4]

∞ Life expectancy. A study[5] in 2016 reviewed all-cause mortality for 29,518 women and explored the differences in causes of death according to sun exposure. The study results were: *'The mortality rate amongst avoiders of sun exposure was approximately twofold higher compared with the highest sun exposure group.'*

Junk light

Unfortunately, all light is not created equal, and light has positive and negative impacts on your body depending on the time of day and the types of light you are exposed to.

There was no artificial light until the light bulb was invented in 1879 and people would rise with the sun, they would wind down for bed by the light of a candle or fire, and sleep when the sun set. It's a beautiful feeling when you step into a room full of candles because it's relaxing and makes your body instantly loosen up. During the day, they would spend long periods of time outside soaking up the sunshine without sunscreen.

Today, it's a completely different life; people wake up in the morning to catch the commuter train while it's dark and they sit under artificial lights all day staring at a screen. If they are lucky, they may get a glimpse of sunlight during lunchtime, and then at night they sit in front of a TV, computer, tablet or smartphone. Is there any wonder that the rate of eye-related problems is spiralling out of control?[6]

As technology has moved into a world of energy efficiency, the much-loved halogen lights have been replaced with LED lights. Unfortunately, indoor lighting from LEDs and screens produces too much artificial blue light. Blue light is known to cause harm by damaging the retina in your eyes and a study conducted in 2018[7] confirmed that blue light exposure is toxic to the eye and results in macular degeneration, a leading cause of blindness in the USA.

Your body wasn't designed to process blue light after dark and LED lights contain a lot of blue light, so you're telling your body that it's continuously 12pm (noon) and it therefore stops production of essential hormones.

> **EXERCISE: Avoid junk light at night.**
>
> Tonight, try to avoid all junk light for at least one hour before you go to bed and see if it makes a difference to the quality of your sleep. This is much easier if you have a device to monitor your sleep but if you don't just notice how you feel when you wake up. Avoiding junk light means, turning down the lights in your home, especially LED bulbs, limited TV and no screens (phones, tablets and laptops).

Irlen Syndrome

Helen Irlen is the founder of the Irlen Institute, investigating the Irlen Syndrome, ® and has pioneered research into the impact that light has on the body. There is too much junk light around because of modern technology, and to make it worse people are often performing more visually intensive activities under artificial lighting. White light (visible light) comprises all the colours of the rainbow, and there are specific wavelengths visible that for some people act as static on their brains. The mind works hard to process the information from the static and it takes up a lot of energy in doing so.

This causes stress to your eyes and brain which can trigger a series of symptoms that impacts your attention, concentration and performance. It can even manifest itself as dizziness, headaches, migraines, nausea, tiredness and sleepiness.

There is a specific test that can be taken so that you can work out the frequencies of light that your body responds best to.

While in California at a conference, I took a test for basic Irlen screening. With a turquoise tint over a piece of white paper I felt it was much easier to read the text.

If you discover that you do have Irlen Syndrome, then you can buy tints for your glasses which will make working under artificial light much more comfortable. Even if people don't have symptoms, many live their lives unaware of this, and how they interpret light and how they feel becomes their new norm. It's not until they experience something different that they realise they have more energy.

Irlen Syndrome is controversial and despite the nay-sayers there are many advocates who claim it's made a massive difference to their lives. The Irlen Institute openly states that they see many people who have been misdiagnosed as having ADHD or dyslexia but have Irlen Syndrome.

Is ultraviolet light bad for you?

Ultraviolet light is split into three components:

1. UV-A – accounts for 95% of the UV light that hits the Earth's surface and it penetrates the deepest layers of the skin.

2. UV-B – cannot penetrate beyond the superficial layers of the skin.

3. UV-C – is the shortest wavelength of light and the most dangerous. Fortunately, UVC is filtered out by the Earth's ozone layer, so it doesn't reach the surface.

Both UV-A and UV-B have been heavily associated with skin cancers, so it's important to treat sunlight with the respect it deserves. However, we are bombarded with advice from the media and the medical community to bathe ourselves in sunscreen and protect our eyes from UV rays, but it's having a detrimental impact on our biology. For example, wearing a sunscreen with a sun protection factor of thirty reduces vitamin D synthesis in the skin by more than 95%.[8] Vitamin D is critically important to bone strength, increasing the immune system, regulating kidney function and regulating blood pressure.

When my clients have a basic blood panel taken, around 50% of them have low vitamin D levels. You need to ensure that you get enough exposure to direct sunlight on your skin, preferably in the early morning or late afternoon when it's not at its strongest.

> **MYTH:** Sunscreen with sun protection factor of fifty is all the protection I need.
>
> **TRUTH:** This isn't true because rates of melanoma mortality have tripled for men and doubled for women over the past sixty years,[9] so sunscreen alone isn't the magic bullet. So, what is? I'm not bashing sunscreen because I use it myself, but it can give a false sense of security and good old common sense needs to prevail. You should stay out of the sun when it's at its strongest and cover up. Like anything, it's the dosage that matters.

When using sunscreen, here is what to look out for:

1. Look for good quality toxin-free products ® with a good SPF value.

2. Avoid spray sunscreen because it contains harmful inhalants and doesn't adequately cover the skin.

3. Don't believe any sunscreen that claims it can protect above SPF 50, it's just a marketing gimmick and has been banned in Europe.

Healing power of infrared light

Infrared light has some amazing benefits but is still little known and hasn't hit the mainstream public. There are three types of infrared light:

1. Near-infrared (IR-A)

2. Mid-infrared (IR-B)

3. Far-infrared (IR-C)

Infrared energy is absorbed by photoreceptors in the cell, triggering a series of metabolic events, increasing blood flow and delivering oxygen and nutrients. Inflammation and pain are reduced, and rejuvenation is stimulated.

CASE STUDY: How infrared light can help.
Here are a few examples of how infrared light has helped:

∞ One day I foolishly performed some exercises at home and didn't do them correctly resulting in a very sore neck. This then spread out to shoulder pain, and I fell into a cycle of each shoulder becoming sore, then my neck. I wasn't sleeping well, and my work was suffering. I then recalled that I had an infrared light at home. I used the light twice on my neck and shoulders for no more than twenty minutes, and the next day the pain subsided massively. Within three days it had gone entirely.

∞ My sister suffers terribly with insect bites; she has a strong reaction to them, her leg swells up, so she has a club foot, and invariably she ends up hobbling around and on a course of antibiotics. Using infrared light on the insect bite resolves the swelling and itching within two or three twenty-minute sessions.

∞ When I suffered from a concussion in early 2018, I used infrared light to speed up the healing process, resulting in my stitches being removed in six rather than nine days. They should have been removed on day four or five because the healing process had accelerated that much.

A 2018 study[10] looked at the impact that photo biomodulation (red or near-infrared light) has on the mitochondria, which they identified as the primary site of light absorption in mammalian cells and concluded that *'photobiomodulation has a marked effect on stem cells and this is proposed to operate via the mitochondria redox signalling'*.

Infrared light does not produce heat but causes a biological reaction and can burn you if not used correctly. Therefore, please proceed with caution, don't fall asleep with a light on your body and don't use it on your head unless you know what you are doing.

There are many infrared devices available on the market for purchase ®, and each of the infrared light frequencies has varying degrees of beneficial properties. I use a light at home with wavelengths of 650 nanometres and 850 nanometres in a single unit ®.

Light and your day

Light impacts your circadian rhythms which trigger hormone release in your body, so you need to make sure you are getting the right kind of light at the correct time of day. The following is a guide for what light you should be looking to be exposed to and what to avoid during a twenty-four-hour cycle:

Morning – in the morning you want the brighter light to tell your body that it's time to wake up so that your melatonin production stops and your cortisol production starts to raise your energy for the day ahead. It's best to get this from sunlight because you also get the benefits of UV and infrared light. If it's winter or not a sunny day, then the next best thing is white light such as a 500-watt halogen light. You can also use a device that shines bright light into your brain and I use this on dark winter mornings Ⓡ.

During the day – this is difficult when you can't control the lighting in your environment, especially where there is a lot of artificial lighting. To keep your circadian rhythms in sync, go for a walk outside or set up a full-spectrum light Ⓡ on your desk. Another option is that when indoors you wear a pair of glasses that block out the junk light Ⓡ. People have reported that by wearing these glasses, they have as much as 30% more energy.

Night-time – when the sun goes down you want to block as much blue light as possible because your body still thinks it's daytime and doesn't switch on your melatonin production. This is the primary reason why people aren't getting as much deep sleep anymore. Once the sun starts to set, slowly dim down your lights. At night you should:

∞ Switch to amber or red bulbs, which have no blue spectrum Ⓡ

∞ Wear blue-blocking glasses at night Ⓡ

∞ Stop staring at bright screens for two hours before bed

∞ Tape over any LEDs in your bedroom and install a blackout curtain Ⓡ

Summary

Sunshine is critically important to your energy levels because it provides you with ultraviolet, visible and infrared light. These spectrums have different positive effects on your body, and unfortunately, people aren't getting enough sunlight anymore. We are spending most of our time under artificial lights and staring at screens which interrupts our circadian rhythms; reducing your exposure to junk light will give you a significant energy boost. Irlen Syndrome is where your brain has problems processing wavelengths of visible light, and it acts like static to your brain and depletes your energy. Finally, the power of infrared light is only just being discovered by science, and its potential for recovery and overall health is likely to be a significant game changer.

Your actions:

- ∞ Ask yourself the question: are you getting enough sunshine and what can you do to get more during your day?

- ∞ Where are you exposed to junk light in your life and what can you do to avoid it?

- ∞ Pick up high-quality sunscreen ®

- ∞ Purchase blue-blocking glasses ®

- ∞ Purchase an infrared light ®

- ∞ Get screened for Irlen Syndrome ®

Part 3 of this book brings all the actions together in an easy-to-follow checklist.

References

1   Lambert, G. W., Reid, C., Kaye, D., Jennings, G. L., & Esler, M. D. (2002). Effect of sunlight and season on serotonin turnover in the brain. *The Lancet*, 360(9348), 1840–1842. PMID: 12480364 – DOI: 10.1016/S0140-6736(02)11737-5

2   Yu, C., Fitzpatrick, A., Cong, D., Yao, C., Yoo, J., Turnbull, A.,& Astier, A. L. (2017). Nitric oxide induces human CLA+ CD25+ Foxp3+ regulatory T cells with skin-homing potential. *Journal of Allergy and Clinical Immunology*, 140(5), 1441–1444. PMID: 28601680 – DOI: 10.1016/J.JACI.2017.05.023

3   Slusher, T. M., Vreman, H. J., Olusanya, B. O., Wong, R. J., Brearley, A. M., Vaucher, Y. E., & Stevenson, D. K. (2014). Safety and efficacy of filtered sunlight in treatment of jaundice in African neonates. *Pediatrics*, 133(6), e1568–74. PMID: 24864170 – DOI: 10.1542/PEDS.2013-3500

4   Zhang, P., & Wu, M. X. (2017). A clinical review of phototherapy for psoriasis. *Lasers in medical science*, 33(1), 173–180. PMID: 29067616 – DOI: 10.1007/S10103-017-2360-1

5   Lindqvist, P. G., Epstein, E., Landin-Olsson, M., Ingvar, C., Nielsen, K., Stenbeck, M., & Olsson H. (2014). Avoidance of sun exposure is a risk factor for all-cause mortality: results from the Melanoma in Southern Sweden cohort. *Journal Internal Medicine*, 276(1), 77–86. PMID: 24697969 – DOI: 10.1111/JOIM.12251

6   Fricke, T. R., Jong, M., Naidoo, K. S., Sankaridurg, P., Naduvilath, T. J., Ho, S. M., Wong, T. Y., … Resnikoff, S. (2018). Global prevalence of visual impairment associated with myopic macular degeneration and temporal trends from 2000 through 2050: systematic review, meta-analysis and modelling. *The British Journal of Ophthalmology*, 102(7), 855–862. PMID: 29699985 – DOI: 10.1136/BJOPHTHALMOL-2017-311266

7   Ratnayake, K., Payton, J. L., Lakmal, O. H., & Karunarathne, A. (2018). Blue light excited retinal intercepts cellular signaling. *Scientific reports*, 8(1), 10207. PMID: 29976989 – DOI: 10.1038/S41598-018-28254-8

8   Nair, R., & Maseeh, A. (2012). Vitamin D: The "sunshine" vitamin. *Journal of pharmacology & pharmacotherapeutics*, 3(2), 118–26. PMID: 22629085. Retrieved from www.jpharmacol.com/article.asp?issn=0976-500X;year=2012;volume=3;issue=2;spage=118;epage=126;aulast=Nair

9   Geller, A. C., Clapp, R. W., Sober, A. J., Gonsalves, L., Mueller, L., Christiansen, C. L., Shaikh, W., … Miller, D. R. (2013). Melanoma epidemic: an analysis of six decades of data from the Connecticut Tumor Registry. *Journal of clinical oncology : official journal of the American Society of Clinical Oncology*, 31(33), 4172–8. PMID: 24043747 – DOI: 10.1200/JCO.2012.47.3728

10 Hamblin, M. R. (2018). Mechanisms and Mitochondrial Redox Signaling in Photobiomodulation. *Photochemistry and photobiology*, 94(2), 199-212. PMID: 29164625 – DOI: 10.1111/PHP.12864

CHAPTER NINE

NOT ALL WATER IS EQUAL

Water is the driving force of all Nature.
LEONARDO DA VINCI

In this chapter you will discover:

- ∞ How to stay hydrated during the day

- ∞ Why tap water may not be as good for you as you think it is

- ∞ The power of adding molecular hydrogen to your water

- ∞ How to manage drinking alcohol

Remember to look out for the recommended resources symbol ®.

Staying hydrated

Around 55–60% of your body is water, and 80% of your brain is water, so it's essential to keep hydrated. A study showed that if you are just 2% dehydrated, attention, memory and physical performance are impaired.[1]

It seems like a simple thing to achieve, yet so many people find it difficult to take on enough fluids during the day. They run from task to task, and before they know it, it's the end of the day, and they haven't drunk enough water.

MYTH: **If my urine is dark, then I must be dehydrated.**

TRUTH: This isn't strictly true although it could be an indicator. If your urine is dark, it could be related to other factors such as your vitamin supplementation or your diet. If you don't go to the bathroom very often, then you're probably not drinking enough water, and if you're going every five minutes, then you've probably had too much water.

The recommended amount of water per day is three litres. The most important part of staying hydrated is to have a container that you always keep with you and holds roughly 500ml ⑱ of water. Think about the times during your day where you can anchor drinking 500ml of water but not in one go. Here are some ideas:

∞ When you first wake up

∞ When you arrive at the office/before you start work

∞ When you come home from school drop-off or work

∞ Before you have lunch

If you can find three times per day to anchor drinking 500ml of water, then you're already 50% of the way there. There are many apps ⑱ for your phone that track your water consumption and send you reminders to make sure you have drunk enough.

Cellular hydration

Drinking the recommended three litres of water a day doesn't necessarily mean that the water is making its way to your cells if you are urinating it straight out. In Chapter 1, we covered the Krebs cycle which enables mitochondria to produce energy. Cellular water is a key component of the Krebs cycle and if you don't have enough water, then your mitochondria can't make enough energy.

Using a specialised device, you can measure something called your phase angle, which is a measurement of how well the cell membranes are functioning and how well hydrated your cells are. There are two elements to the phase angle:

∞ Reactance: reflects the body cell mass

∞ Resistance: reflects the water or fluid at a cellular level

A phase angle of 6 to 8 is considered good with 10 being ideal. A phase angle of 3.5 is where death occurs.

Zach Bush MD is a triple board-certified physician with expertise in Internal Medicine, Endocrinology and Metabolism, and Hospice/Palliative care. In an interview[2] on cellular hydration with Dr Joseph Mercola he stated:

> *'Interestingly, all our cancer patients tend to come in around 4.5 or below, which is interesting because it suggests, from a hydration standpoint cancer doesn't happen until you're so dry that you're nearly dead. In this way, cancer is not a disease that pops out of anywhere.'*

A 2018 review[3] in the *European Journal of Clinical Nutrition* conducted a systematic review of existing scientific papers on the link between phase angle and mortality. It concluded that:

'Phase angle seems to be a good indicator for mortality in many clinical situations and can be used in screening individuals prone to this outcome.'

To improve your phase angle and get hydrated at a cellular level you need to:

- ∞ Supplement electrolytes. Common electrolytes are calcium, chloride, magnesium, potassium and sodium. You probably are getting enough sodium, chloride and calcium each day, but you may want to consider supplementing with potassium and magnesium.

- ∞ Get more fibre. Vegetables are packed with fibre which absorbs water and then carries it through your bloodstream to your cells.

Tap water

There have been many cases in the UK and USA where drinking water has been contaminated. In particular, the 2014 water crisis in Flint, Michigan where 100,000 residents, including 8,000 children under the age of six, were exposed to high levels of lead in their drinking water. Since this time, dozens of other cities in the USA have reported similar issues.

Congress in the USA banned lead pipes thirty years ago, but millions of older ones remain and leach lead into the water during repairs or changes in the chemistry of the water. Similarly, the UK banned lead pipes in the 1970s, but many are still underground or are inside older homes.

'The DWI (Drinking Water Inspectorate) says that all UK tap water is safe to drink and that they conduct millions of tests per year to guarantee the best water quality. These standards are based on European legislation and science from the World Health Organization. In 2014, water companies carried out over 4.5 million tests of water for around fifty different chemical and microbiological substances.'

Fifty different chemicals and microbiological substances are a fraction of what will exist in water, and all fifty chemicals and microbial materials can exist in the water but have to be below set thresholds, which are considered to be within a safe tolerance for humans. These include mercury, aluminium, arsenic, benzene, lead and pesticides. Chlorine is also added to your drinking water to keep it disinfected and to keep the water clean. When chlorine meets your stomach, it is going to do its job and kill bacteria.

I'm not knocking the water companies; it's incredibly challenging to be able to supply drinking water to the country and have it completely clean. In *Resources,* I have shared the 'Prescribed/Specification Concentration or Values as listed in the Water Supply (Water Quality) Regulations 2016' ®.

Will the low level of these substances damage my health in the long-term? Who knows, but I prefer not to take the risk when I'm drinking four litres of water a day. In researching this book, I came across the following interesting facts on the UK drinking water supply:

∞ Lead pipes were banned in the UK in the 1970s, and many water companies are undergoing a process to replace all lead pieces. If you live in a house that was built post-1970, then it is less likely you will have lead pipes carrying water to your home. However, it's still worth checking.

∞ In the UK, 10% of the drinking water has fluoride added to it to help prevent tooth decay. That's a good thing, right? Unfortunately not. Adding fluoride to water has been banned in many European Countries, because it's toxic and an endocrine disruptor.[4]

∞ According to a report by the Guardian newspaper, in 2011, the slug poison metaldehyde was found in one in eight of England's sources of drinking water.[5]

Whether you drink tap water or not is a personal decision. I prefer to drink filtered water, with my next preference being glass bottled water. Plastic bottles are not always a better alternative because they are bad for the environment and even though the recycling rates are high, plastic is finding its way into waterways and the sea, where it degrades over time and enters the food system through fish.

MYTH: Plastic bottles can be reused.
TRUTH: Reusing soft plastic bottles is not good for your health because the plastic chemicals can leach into the water if they are exposed to heat or have been sat around for a long time.

Water filters

Water filters are commonplace in many homes either because people dislike the taste of tap water or they are looking to mitigate the risk of what may be in their water supply. There are many different water filter options available.

The most affordable option is the water filter jug Ⓡ, where you pour water into the top of the jug, and it then passes through a carbon filter, and you keep the water in the fridge. It's not the most convenient way to filter your water, but it does do a decent job of removing lead, perfluorocarbons (PCBs), pesticides, herbicides, chlorine, some bacteria and some parasites. You may also find that if your refrigerator has a water dispenser, it may well run it through a similar carbon filter. If you want to take it up a level, then you can purchase a much larger carbon block filter Ⓡ, and filter all water coming into your house. This is a much larger undertaking, and you are likely to need the help of a qualified plumber.

Reverse osmosis filters Ⓡ do a much better job of removing impurities from water and are considered the gold standard because they remove all the heavy metals, bacteria and parasites that carbon misses. You can have them fitted under your sink, surface mounted or as part of your house supply. The downside with reverse osmosis filters is that due to the way they operate, they can waste a lot of water. For example, for every four litres of water produced they waste at least one litre.

Molecular hydrogen water

Molecular hydrogen (H2) is a tasteless and odourless gas that is now known to be a potent antioxidant, neutralising free radicals that contribute to disease development, inflammation and ageing. Hydrogen is unique because of its ability to activate the Nrf2 (Nuclear factor erythroid-derived 2) pathways inside your body which signal the production of glutathione, antioxidant enzymes or survival genes. Nrf2 is a powerful protein that is latent within your cells that doesn't function until released by a Nrf2 activator.

Hydrogen is the smallest of molecules, having just two atoms, making it an ideal antioxidant. It's thought that H2 may be the only antioxidant that can make its way inside the mitochondria. It can then work deep inside the cell to neutralise free radicals and reduce oxidative stress. There are no downsides because when hydrogen neutralises a free radical, the by-product is water.

The easiest way to get H2 into your system is to drop molecular hydrogen tablets **ⓡ** into water and then drink it. The hydrogen will enter your bloodstream and then be transported to all areas of your body.

Molecular hydrogen has been known to science for a couple of hundred years, but its profile rose rapidly following a study published in *Nature Medicine*[6] which demonstrated its antioxidant properties. Since then there have been hundreds of reviews and articles showing molecular hydrogen's benefits.

Benefits of hydrogen water include:

∞ Helps to prevent diabetes. A 2008 study[7] of thirty people with type 2 diabetes (T2DM) who drank four cups of hydrogen water every day for eight weeks concluded that:

'these results suggest that supplementation with hydrogen-rich water may have a beneficial role in the prevention of T2DM and insulin resistance'.

∞ Helps to prevent cancer. Molecular hydrogen's powerful antioxidant properties mean that it eats up free radicals which, as you learned in Part 1 of this book, cause oxidative stress and cancer.[8]

∞ Reduces symptoms of rheumatoid arthritis. Arthritis is an inflammatory condition, and molecular hydrogen is effective in reducing inflammation.[9]

Drinking alcohol

Alcohol is a sure-fire way to wreck your performance, but sometimes it's enjoyable and worth taking the hit. When you are twenty-one years of age it is easy, but as you get older, balancing fun and entertainment with performance the next day is tricky.

Five ways to minimise the hangover and stay at peak performance:

1. Take two activated charcoal tablets Ⓡ before you drink any alcohol. Toxins from the alcohol will bind to the charcoal and pass through you rather than poison your mitochondria. It is even better if you can take additional activated charcoal tablets in between drinks.

2. When you've finished drinking, supplement with glutathione Ⓡ. It is the body's master antioxidant and what your liver uses to process alcohol. When your liver runs out of glutathione, it causes liver damage.

3. When drinking, try and stay away from beer and red wine as they contain more toxins than other options. It's best to drink good quality vodka, gin, white wine or sparkling wine. The distillation process for vodka and gin produces a drink which is purer than the other options. If you love your wine, look at biodynamic or natural wines ® as these are made the 'old way' and therefore have fewer toxins and sulfites.

4. Be intentional, don't fall into the trap of 'it will be ok'. If you have a late night, be intentional with your morning routine, prioritise your sleep and drink plenty of water before going to bed.

5. Take a PQQ / CoQ10 supplement ® to help repair your damaged mitochondria and provide you with a boost of energy that will clear your brain fog.

> **CASE STUDY:** Alcohol is toxic, so you shouldn't drink too much, but it's become so ingrained in many cultures it becomes difficult to avoid for some people, especially where alcohol ties in with work functions. I remember one of my prospective clients looking at me in disbelief when I told him I have a hack so that he can avoid a hangover. He went out and purchased the charcoal tablets and gluta-thione and sent me a message a few days later gobsmacked that he had woken up without a hangover. He then went on to become a client.

Summary

Staying hydrated is important because even a small decrease in hydration can have a significant impact on your performance. Try and aim for three to four litres a day and drink water anchored to specific times in your day. Most countries in the world now have access to drinking water in their homes, and your quality of water is endorsed against the World Health Organization's standards. My personal view is that the standards aren't good enough and there are still too many heavy metals, pesticides, chemicals and hormones in your drinking water. Adding molecular hydrogen to water has some fantastic health benefits, and it's something that I use every day to keep my health and performance on track. When drinking alcohol, you can mitigate some of the effects by supplementing with activated charcoal ® and glutathione ®.

Your actions:

- ∞ Purchase a drinks container to enable you to get more fluids in each day ®

- ∞ Follow the guidelines on how to stay hydrated by anchoring your drinking to specific events in your day

- ∞ Do your research on tap water and make an intentional decision

- ∞ Purchase molecular hydrogen tablets and take them every day to enjoy the performance and health-span benefits ®

- ∞ Purchase activated charcoal and glutathione for your next night out ®

Part 3 of this book brings all the actions together in an easy-to-follow checklist.

References

1   Wittbrodt, M. T., & Millard-Stafford, M. (2018). Dehydration Impairs Cognitive Performance: A Meta-analysis. *Medicine and science in sports and exercise*, 50(11), 2360–2368. PMID: 29933347 – DOI: 10.1249/MSS.0000000000001682

2   Mercola, J. (2018, May 06). Hydration Is About More Than Just Drinking Water – How to Hydrate at the Cellular Level to Improve Health and Longevity. Retrieved from https://articles.mercola.com/sites/articles/archive/2018/05/06/how-to-hydrate-at-the-cellular-level.aspx

3   Garlini, L. M., Alves, F. D., Ceretta, L. B., Perry, I. S., Souza, G. C., & Clausell, N. O. (2018). Phase angle and mortality: a systematic review. *European Journal of Clinical Nutrition.* PMID: 29695763 – DOI: 10.1038/S41430-018-0159-1

4   Peckham, S., Lowery, D., & Spencer, S. (2015). Are fluoride levels in drinking water associated with hypothyroidism prevalence in England? A large observational study of GP practice data and fluoride levels in drinking water. *Journal of Epidemiology & Community Health*, 69(7), 619–624. PMID: 25714098 – DOI: 10.1136/JECH-2014-204971

5   Mathiesen, K. (2013 July,10). Slug poison found in one in eight of England's drinking water sources. *The Guardian.* Retrieved from www.theguardian.com/environment/2013/jul/10/slug-poison-drinking-water-metaldehyde

6   Ohsawa, I., Ishikawa, M., Takahashi, K., Watanabe, M., Nishimaki, K. et al (2007). Hydrogen acts as a therapeutic antioxidant by selectively reducing cytotoxic oxygen radicals. *Nature Medicine*, 13(6), 688–694. PMID: 17486089 – DOI: 10.1038/NM1577

7   Kajiyama, S., Hasegawa, G., Asano, M., Hosoda, H., Fukui, M., Nakamura, N., & Adachi, T. (2008). Supplementation of hydrogen-rich water improves lipid and glucose metabolism in patients with type 2 diabetes or impaired glucose tolerance. *Nutrition Research*, 28(3), 137–143. PMID: 19083400 – DOI: 10.1016/J.NUTRES.2008.01.008

8   Asada, R., Kageyama, K., Tanaka, H., Matsui, H., Kimura, M., Saitoh, Y., & Miwa, N. (2010). Antitumor effects of nano-bubble hydrogen-dissolved water are enhanced by coexistent platinum colloid and the combined hyperthermia with apoptosis-like cell death. *Oncology reports*, 24(6), 1463–1470. PMID: 21042740 – DOI:10.1016/J.JPHOTOBIOL.2011.09.006

9   Ishibashi, T., Sato, B., Rikitake, M., Seo, T., Kurokawa, R., Hara, Y., & Nagao, T. (2012). Consumption of water containing a high concentration of molecular hydrogen reduces oxidative stress and disease activity in patients with rheumatoid arthritis: an open-label pilot study. *Medical gas research*, 2(1), 27. PMID: 23031079 – DOI: 10.1186/2045-9912-2-27

CHAPTER TEN

TOXINS WILL KILL YOUR PERFORMANCE

> *Illness is the result of improper removal of toxins from the body. Oxygen is the vital factor which assists the body in removing toxins.*
>
> **ED MCCABE**

In this chapter, you will discover:

- ∞ Why you should minimise your exposure to toxins

- ∞ Where toxins hide and the sources of environmental toxins

- ∞ How to effectively detoxify

Remember to look out for the recommended resources symbol ⓡ.

Toxins are a fact of life

The world of health and self-development is focused on what you should be doing, but it doesn't focus so much on what you shouldn't be doing and what you should be avoiding. Toxins are all around you, every single day, and it's now an unavoidable fact of life; you are living in a synthetic soup that shows no sign of getting better. Toxicity in the environment is no doubt leading to inflammation and disease but it's also having a significant impact on the sperm count of males, and over the past four decades, sperm counts have dropped 52%.[1]

MYTH: **Toxins can only enter my body through the air that I breathe and what I eat or drink.**

TRUTH: Toxins not only enter your body through breathing but also through your skin. The skin is the body's largest organ and is very absorbent. A study conducted by the University of Ottawa in 2017[2] showed that firefighters absorbed harmful chemicals through their skin while fighting fires despite wearing breathing apparatus.

When you think of toxins, the first thought you probably have is of large city pollution, the common sight of smog filling the air of a sprawling city and people walking around with masks covering their mouths. There is no doubt that these air pollutants are not good for you, but there are many other hidden toxins that are affecting your energy and performance. It's not only the air you breathe but the things you touch, what you eat and even what you see and hear.

You are unique, and we will each process toxins in different ways, some people will feel the exposure of certain toxins more than others. However, it's fair to say that even if you don't feel a negative impact from exposure to toxins, it's going to be impacting your performance. It's always best to minimise your exposure.

Toxins impact your mitochondria,[3] deplete your energy, disturb your sleep and affect your mood. Here is an initial set of environmental toxins that you should look to minimise your exposure to:

∞ Toxic mould

∞ Glyphosate

∞ Skin and cleaning products

∞ Electromagnetic frequencies

If you search for any of the above, you will find a mixed bag of comments on the internet. On one side you have a set of people who are super sensitive to some of these toxins and on the other side the 'Big Companies' who make millions by selling their products.

Toxic mould

I remember being a student and my friends and I would grow mould in our coffee cups to see who could get the largest culture. Mould can be very beneficial. For example, the penicillium mould produces the antibiotic penicillin and is considered a wonder drug because it was used to treat infections from wounds during World War II and saved many lives.

Most mould is non-toxic. However, some species of mould produce mycotoxins which are harmful to humans. Mycotoxin exposure is going to impact everybody to some degree, and the extent will partly depend on your genetics. Some individuals are super sensitive to mycotoxins and can become very ill and be misdiagnosed as having depression, Lyme disease, fibromyalgia and chronic fatigue syndrome.

If you have exposure to mycotoxins you may experience:

∞ Brain fog

∞ Cognitive dysfunction

∞ Mood issues

∞ High levels of inflammation

∞ Fatigue

∞ Weight gain

About one in four people have a sensitivity to mould, which you'll typically find where there is excessive moisture, such as kitchens, bathrooms and where water leaks have previously occurred. You will also find that some foods are particularly susceptible to toxic mould and I have included a list of them below. A client of mine had toxic mould issues that were so bad that he developed a cough whenever he travelled on the London underground.

As long as there has been life on Earth, there has been a continual battle between mould and bacteria. As your mitochondria are so similar to bacteria, it is no surprise that exposure to toxic mould has a negative impact on your energy and performance.

The solution:

∞ Ensure that you have plenty of ventilation in
   your home.

∞ Check all pipework on a regular basis for water leaks. Where you do have a mould problem, have it properly treated, and the root cause addressed.

∞ Ensure there is no visible sign of mould in your food and take note that most of the time mould can be invisible to the human eye. Foods that are susceptible to mould include aged meats, beans, brazil nuts, bread, corn, cheese, chilli spices (high risk), dried fruit, grains (except white rice), oats, peanuts, pistachios (high risk of mould but very good for you if they are a clean source) and pre-ground black pepper (high risk).

Pesticides

Glyphosate is the chemical that you will commonly find in the weed killer that you spray over your garden or drive to kill off any unwanted plants. It's effective and has become the primary source for killing off plants.

Glyphosate has a fascinating history as it was one of a blend of herbicides called Agent Orange and was used in the Vietnam War to clear the land, enabling the troops to infiltrate the dense forests. Unfortunately, as the war progressed, they discovered that Agent Orange was responsible for many deaths through cancer, so they stopped spraying. Since then glyphosate has been patented many times as an antibiotic, anti-fungal and anti-viral. It is extremely useful in killing all organic material, not just plant material.

The shocking thing about glyphosate is that in many parts of the world, crops are sprayed with it as a pre-harvest application to ensure the wheat ripens evenly. Glyphosate is also sprayed on genetically modified crops to ease the harvesting process. Genetically modified crops such as corn and soy are modified to withstand the toxic load. Not only is glyphosate being sprayed on the food you consume, but it's also sprayed through the air, which then makes its way into the water system because glyphosate is water soluble. Glyphosate is not only toxic, but it also impacts your gut microbes[4] and kills the bacteria in the soil.

The International Agency for Research on Cancer called the chemical 'probably carcinogenic',[5] but others have said it's safe to use. The European Food Safety Authority (EFSA) says glyphosate is unlikely to cause cancer in humans.[6] However, in a 2017 vote to renew the licence of glyphosate, nine EU member states[7] voted against a 5-year extension.

In August 2018 a California jury found Monsanto liable in a lawsuit filed by a school groundskeeper, Dewayne Johnson, who alleged the company's glyphosate-based weed-killers caused his cancer. The jury awarded Dewayne Johnson $289 million in damages.[8]

The solution:

- ∞ Go through your garden shed, throw away anything that contains glyphosate and use a natural weed killer, such as your hands or a solution of salt and vinegar Ⓡ.

- ∞ Eat organic whenever possible. The list of foods being sprayed with glyphosate is proliferating and is too long to list here Ⓡ.

Cosmetics

Your skin is very absorbent, and it's your body's largest organ, so it is an effective way for toxins to make their way inside of you. I'm not sure who I first heard say this, but as a rule of thumb 'if I won't put it in my mouth, then I won't put it on my skin'. I stopped using all creams, soaps, shampoo and deodorant. You're probably thinking 'yuck, he must walk around smelly all of the time'. I've asked my wife, and she says I smell fine.

The thing is that when you clean up your diet and your toxic load is low, you don't suffer from body odour as much, and your farts stop smelling. You don't need to use much of, or any, chemical products. I do use some shampoo ⑧ and body wash products ⑧, but they are natural, and while they wouldn't taste good, I could eat them. I also use a toxin-free sunscreen ⑧ when I go away on holiday.

The same goes for cleaning products at home, some of them can be extremely toxic and people often clean without gloves or a face mask. Wherever possible, wear a mask, gloves and seek out products that don't have a high toxic load.

The solution:

∞ Source low toxicity products ⑧

∞ Wear adequate protection when using cleaning products

EMFs

Electromagnetic Frequencies (EMFs) are an extremely contro-versial subject and one that I've personally taken a while to come to terms with. I'm a self-confessed technology geek and a huge fan of the Internet of Things, quantified self and technology-enabled homes.

The increase in Wi-Fi and Bluetooth-enabled devices has escalated so quickly that scientists don't know what the long-term effects may be. Wi-Fi is pervasive and has become part of life; it's always there and all around us at home and work. As the quantified self and wearable tech movements continue to grow exponentially, there will be more SIM card-enabled devices mounted on people's bodies.

Examples of EMF devices are:

- ∞ Microwave ovens

- ∞ Mobile phone/SIM card-enabled devices

- ∞ Wi-Fi routers

- ∞ Laptop/tablets

- ∞ Cordless land-line phones

- ∞ Technology-enabled sensors, light bulbs and thermostats

CASE STUDY: In my home, I have four Wi-Fi routers, various devices, thirty technology-enabled light bulbs, thermostats and doorbells. I have more than average, but this kind of setup will be commonplace soon. I used an EMF reader ⓚ in my house, and this is what I found.

The readings in the middle of my house were: 0.282 mw/m².

The readings in my office where I work were: 4.145 mw/m².

Just by making a few tweaks to my environment I was able to reduce the readings in my office down to: 0.09 mw/m².

The two factors with EMF exposure to consider are:

∞ Proximity: how close are you to the EMF device? The further away, the better.

∞ Duration: how long are you exposed for?

That's why I don't think it's a good idea to be wearing SIM card-enabled devices on your body because the signal is going to be strong and you're wearing them continuously.

The scientific evidence is unclear about whether electromagnetic frequencies have a negative impact on the human body and disrupt your mitochondria. Scientists have confirmed that EMFs do not cook your cells, as people speculated in the 1990s, but what they do is activate something called voltage-gated calcium channels (VGCCs)[9] which are in the outer membranes of your cells. When activated, they allow calcium into your cells, increasing both nitric oxide and superoxide, which is a potent oxidant stressor.

Solutions:

- ∞ Minimise your exposure to EMFs by keeping your phone in aeroplane mode when it's in your pocket

- ∞ Put as much distance between yourself and your Wi-Fi router as possible

- ∞ Put any wearable devices on aeroplane mode when not required to sync data

- ∞ Consider taking molecular hydrogen to help mop up any free radicals ®

What else to watch out for?

I could probably write a whole book on toxins, so here is a list of other toxins that you may want to research further:

- ∞ Mercury fillings ®

- ∞ Heavy metals

- ∞ Non-stick-coated cookery items ®

- ∞ Air fresheners

- ∞ Bug sprays

- ∞ Petrol station fumes

- ∞ Plastics containing Bisphenol A (BPA) ®

Detoxification

Detoxification is critical to ensure you are removing as much of the waste and junk from your body as possible before it starts to cause a problem. A detoxification process uses your body's natural processes by:

∞ Stimulating the liver to drive toxins out from the body

∞ Elimination of the toxins through the intestines, kidneys and skin

∞ Improving circulation of the blood

The organs that are used to detoxify are the lymph glands, colon, liver, lungs, kidneys and skin. It's a good idea to support these if detoxifying.

The following are the most effective ways to detoxify:

∞ Sauna – Research has proven that an effective way to detoxify is to sweat in a sauna. Sweating can remove lead, cadmium, arsenic and mercury.

∞ Infrared Sauna – Infrared saunas are more useful for detoxification because the infrared heat penetrates deeper into the body and causes a more vigorous sweat.

∞ Exercise – Exercise helps to detoxify the body, but it doesn't have to be full-on and blood pumping. It can be a low-intensity aerobic exercise that gets the body moving and heart pumping such as walking or cycling. This is part of the reasoning behind getting people to walk 10,000 steps a day.

∞ Water – Drink a lot of water per day, preferably three to four litres (Chapter 9). Your kidneys eliminate toxins and waste products from your urine and blood. Around 55 to 60% of your body is water, and 80% of your brain is water, so it's essential to keep hydrated.

∞ Coffee enema ® – It is possible to perform an enema at home to help with detoxification. This flushes out your colon and stimulates your liver to produce glutathione.

∞ Glutathione ® – this is the body's master antioxidant and is fundamental to your ability to detoxify.

Releasing toxins from within your body can be dangerous, so please proceed with care. You need the released toxins to bind to something and then come out of your body. So please be careful with some of the crazy detox protocols on the internet and don't detoxify heavy metals without support from a Functional Medical Practitioner.

When you detox, please make sure you:

1. Supplement with glutathione to support your liver ®

2. Take activated charcoal to help bind the toxins ®

3. Drink plenty of water

Summary

Toxins are an inevitable part of your life, and you cannot avoid them, but you can minimise them. Toxins lead to inflammation in the body which leads to disease, so do everything you can to limit your exposure. You will not be able to eliminate toxins entirely so have a protocol in place to detoxify yourself on a regular basis.

Your actions:

- ∞ Ensure that in your home you have plenty of ventilation

- ∞ Check all pipework on a regular basis for water leaks. Where you do have a mould problem, have it properly treated, and the root cause addressed

- ∞ Ensure there is no visible sign of mould in your food and take note that most of the time mould can be invisible to the human eye

- ∞ Go through your garden shed, throw away anything that contains glyphosate and use a natural weed killer, such as your hands or a solution of salt and vinegar ®

- ∞ Eat organic whenever possible. The list of foods being sprayed with glyphosate is proliferating and is too long to list here ®

- ∞ Minimise your exposure to EMFs by keeping your phone in aeroplane mode when it's in your pocket

- ∞ Move your Wi-Fi router as far away as possible from where you spend most of the time

- ∞ Put any wearable devices on aeroplane mode when not required to sync data

- ∞ Consider taking molecular hydrogen to help mop up any free radicals ®

Part 3 of this book brings all the actions together in an easy-to-follow checklist.

References

1   Levine, H., Jørgensen, N., Martino-Andrade, A., Mendiola, J., Weksler-Derri, D., Mindlis, I., & Swan, S. H. (2017). Temporal trends in sperm count: a systematic review and meta-regression analysis. *Human Reproduction Update*, 23(6), 646–659. PMID: 28981654 – DOI: 10.1093/HUMUPD/DMX022

2   Keir, J. L., Akhtar, U. S., Matschke, D. M., Kirkham, T. L., Chan, H. M., Ayotte, P., ... & Blais, J. M. (2017). Elevated Exposures to Polycyclic Aromatic Hydrocarbons and Other Organic Mutagens in Ottawa Firefighters Participating in Emergency, On-Shift Fire Suppression. *Environmental science & technology*, 51(21), 12745–12755. PMID: 29043785 – DOI: 10.1021/ACS.EST.7B02850

3   Meyer, J. N., Leung, M. C., Rooney, J. P., Sendoel, A., Hengartner, M. O., Kisby, G. E., & Bess, A. S. (2013). Mitochondria as a target of environmental toxicants. *Toxicological sciences : an official journal of the Society of Toxicology*, 134(1), 1–17. PMID: 23629515 – DOI: 10.1093/TOXSCI/KFT102

4   Samsel, A., & Seneff, S. (2013). Glyphosate, pathways to modern diseases II: Celiac sprue and gluten intolerance. *Interdisciplinary toxicology*, 6(4), 159–84. PMID: 24678255 – DOI: 10.2478/INTOX-2013-0026

5   Evaluation of five organophosphate insecticides and herbicides. (2015, March 20). Retrieved from: https://www.iarc.fr/wp-content/uploads/2018/07/MonographVolume112-1.pdf

6   European Food Safety Authority (EFSA) (2015). Conclusion on the peer review of the pesticide risk assessment of the active substance glyphosate. *EFSA Journal*, 13(11), 4302. DOI: 10.2903/J.EFSA.2015.4302

7   European Commission (2017). Summary report of the Appeal Committee – Phytopharmaceuticals – Plant Protection Products – Legislation. Retrieved from https://ec.europa.eu/food/sites/food/files/plant/docs/sc_phyto_20171127_pppl_summary.pdf

8   Levin. S., & Greenfield, P. (2018, Aug 11). Monsanto ordered to pay $289m as jury rules weedkiller caused man's cancer. *The Guardian*. Retrieved from www.theguardian.com/business/2018/aug/10/monsanto-trial-cancer-dewayne-johnson-ruling

9   Pall, M. L. (2013). Electromagnetic fields act via activation of voltage-gated calcium channels to produce beneficial or adverse effects. *Journal of cellular and molecular medicine*, 17(8), 958–965. PMID: 23802593 – DOI:10.1111/JCMM.12088

CHAPTER ELEVEN

FLOOD YOUR BODY WITH OXYGEN

When you feel life is out of focus,
always return to the basic of life.
Breathing. No breath, no life.

MR MIYAGI

In this chapter you will discover:

∞ The reason why and how you breathe is as important as what you eat

∞ How to learn to breathe correctly and learn to breathe through your nose

∞ The breathing techniques to help you in the moment

∞ The importance of Heart Rate Variability training

∞ The benefits of oxygen therapy including EWOT, hyperbaric and ozone

Remember to look out for the recommended resources symbol ®.

Blood oxygen levels

A measurement of oxygen in your blood is called your oxygen saturation level and is often referred to as 'sats'. A device called a pulse oximeter is used to measure your oxygen saturation, and it works by sending infrared light into your finger, toe or earlobe. It's accurate to 2% either way, so if you measure 96%, you could be between 94 and 98%. A normal level is 95 to 100%, and anything below 92% is cause for concern and is referred to as hypoxaemia. When hypoxaemia occurs, symptoms that can arise are rapid heartbeat, shortness of breath, chest pains, confusion and headaches.

Haemoglobin in your red blood cells is responsible for transporting oxygen around your body and each molecule of haemoglobin can hold four oxygen molecules. If you recall in Chapter 1 of this book, oxygen is critical for your mitochondria to produce adenosine triphosphate (ATP). If you don't have enough oxygen in your bloodstream and reaching your cells, then your mitochondria aren't going to be able to create energy as effectively. Having enough oxygen in your bloodstream is critical to your performance.

Breathing correctly

I love the quote at the start of this chapter. When I saw it, I knew I just had to include it. I know Mr Miyagi is a fictional character from *The Karate Kid*, but I love the quote, and I love Mr Miyagi. Breathing isn't something that most people give a great deal of thought to; it's something that you do continually all day, every day. It's the first thing you do when you are born and the last thing you will do when you die. It's critical to life because:

- ∞ Breathing supplies oxygen to the blood which is then carried to the cells throughout the body, where it helps convert nutrients into usable energy in the process of cellular respiration. I covered this in Chapter 1 of this book.

∞ Breathing helps to remove toxins and other harmful substances from your body.

∞ Breathing eliminates carbon dioxide from your body.

So how important is it to breathe in the right way?

Slow, deep and regular breathing leads to a calm mind and body while fast, shallow breathing is an indication of high stress and anxiousness. Most people aren't breathing in the right way because modern life makes them breathe shallow and quickly with their mouths open, during the day and when they sleep.

MYTH: **Deep breaths are best for us.**

TRUTH: So often, we hear the instruction to take a big breath. This doesn't add any more oxygen but does get rid of more carbon dioxide, which contracts your muscles and squeezes the vessels and impacts circulation. You want your breaths to be deep and not detectable.

Most people believe it's good to take big breaths into the lungs, but when your breathing is undetectable, it's a sign that your blood is almost entirely saturated by oxygen.

Normal breathing uses five to eight litres per minute but people with breathing issues will typically breathe at eight to ten litres per minute. Asthmatics' breathing can be ten to fifteen litres per minute.

A useful tool from Buteyko Breathing is the Control Pause[1] because it provides feedback on your breathing volume.

EXERCISE: Control pause.

Rest for ten minutes before starting the exercise.

∞ Take a small breath in through your nose and allow a small breath out through your nose.

∞ Hold your breath. Close your mouth tight and hold your nose with your finger and thumb.

∞ Count the number of seconds until you feel some discomfort and a desire to breathe.

∞ Your inhalation at the end of the breath should be calm. (If your inhalation was a big breath, then you've held your breath for too long.)

∞ Release your nose and breathe.

Control Pause timings are rated as follows:

∞ 40 seconds – very good

∞ 30 seconds – good

∞ 25 – room for improvement

∞ Less than 15 – is a sign of respiratory complaints, sleep disorders or anxiety

Nasal breathing

You have two options when you breathe; either through your nose or your mouth. Many people, when they sleep, exercise or go about their daily routine, rely a lot less on their nose to take in oxygen but instead use their mouths, which results in very shallow breathing. The most apparent impact of breathing through your mouth on a regular basis is snoring. If you wake up in the morning with a parched mouth, then you were breathing through your mouth at night. You should wake up with a slightly moist mouth.

Your nasal passage is much smaller than your mouth, so this gives your lungs extra time to extract the oxygen. Breathing in through the mouth is inefficient, particularly when you exercise, because you need to obtain more oxygen from each breath. Your nose also has a filtration system that takes particles out of the air and kills bacteria and viruses.

Your sinuses play a role in filtering and warming the air as it hits your lungs, which helps to keep harmful bacteria and particles out of your body. They also help to warm the air and produce 25% of your nitric oxide, which promotes healthy dilation of veins and arteries.

Breathing techniques

Practising breathing exercises can help regulate your breathing rate and has many benefits including lowering blood pressure, reducing anxiety, improving sleep and lowering stress.

The following breathing techniques are particularly useful to perform pre-presentation or before difficult meetings.

Box breath

One of the more straightforward exercises which can be done at any time and in any place is the box breath. This will help calm your nervous system during times of stress and help you reset and regain your composure.

EXERCISE: Box breath.

The box breath has four simple stages:

∞ Breathe in for four seconds

∞ Hold your breath for four seconds

∞ Breathe out for four seconds

∞ Hold your breath for four seconds.

∞ And repeat four times.

This is an incredibly simple breathing exercise that will have a significant impact on your performance, especially when you're undergoing stress.

3-4-7 breathing

Another variant on the box breath is 3-4-7 breathing:

EXERCISE: 3-4-7 breathing.

The box breath has four simple stages:

∞ Breathe in for three seconds

∞ Hold for four seconds

∞ Breathe out for seven seconds

∞ Repeat several times in a row

If you're experiencing heavy stress, this will help increase the oxygen flow to your brain and will help calm you down.

Heart Rate Variability (HRV) training

HRV Training is one of the most important things you can do and while I could have included it within the section on breathing techniques, it's so important it needs its own section. You use a device to measure your HRV and then perform breathing exercises and positive thoughts to change your HRV.

HRV is the spacing between your heartbeats rather than how fast your heart beats. When you're relaxed, your parasympathetic and sympathetic nervous system is in balance. When you are stressed, your heart rate is more rhythmic with little or no variability.

For example, if your heart beats at 60 beats per minute and the intervals between your heart beats are:

- ∞ Regular – 1 beat per second, then this signifies a stressed state

- ∞ Variable – 1.02, 0.98, 0.96, 1.03, etc, then this signifies a relaxed state

HRV is a crucial indicator of your emotional state, how well you cope with stressful situations, and if you're in a state of peak performance.[2]

Many of my clients feel pressure from the demands of their business, family, social life, following their interests and living a full life. It's no surprise that stress levels are often running high with the need to balance a personal life with the professional pressures of critical pitches, keynote presentations, back-to-back meetings and looming deadlines.

When you are stressed you've activated your freeze, fight or flight response and you won't be in a high performing state; you will get easily distracted, allow your mind to tell you self-defeating stories and beat yourself up for not doing well enough.

What if you could train yourself to have good HRV and:

∞ Take the stress out of the equation and shift stress-producing emotional states

∞ Access intuition for making better decisions

∞ Increase mental clarity, energy and focus

∞ Release and prevent overwhelm

∞ Boost your resilience

Well, you can – by using an HRV monitor and focusing on positive emotional thoughts, while carrying out controlled breathing exercises you're able to increase your HRV and fundamentally change your response to stress. HRV Training is also an effective way to increase alpha brainwaves (Chapter 14).

Learning to deal with your sympathetic nervous system used to take years of meditation to achieve but now, with HRV Training, this is no longer the case. I use a specific biofeedback device ⓡ with my clients to increase their HRV over a six-week period, and it only takes ten minutes per day. This type of training can have a profound impact on your life and will keep you in a high performing state.

Oxygen therapies

Oxygen therapies are not well studied and are relatively new, but are gaining popularity as an alternative way to reduce inflammation and treat chronic conditions. Don't confuse oxygen therapies with oxygen bars. They have a terrible reputation as quack science and are even touted as harmful, but I have an open mind. However, that's not what I'm covering here. The three types of therapy I'll include are:

1. Exercise with Oxygen Therapy (EWOT)

2. Ozone Therapy

3. Hyperbaric Oxygen Chambers

Exercise with Oxygen Therapy

Exercise with Oxygen Therapy (EWOT), otherwise known as Oxygen Multistep Therapy, has been studied extensively by Manfred von Ardenne, a German scientist. There are very few scientific studies but the therapy has many fans who claim it's helped them overcome health conditions and increased their athletic performance.

To perform EWOT, you exercise in one place while wearing an oxygen mask. The exercises usually performed could be running, using a cross-trainer or cycling. Wearing the oxygen mask enables the body to receive more high-flow rate 'oxygen enriched air' (90% and above) than it would from the room. This, in turn, increases the red blood cells' capability to carry oxygen but also increases oxygen in the blood plasma.

As you age, the amount of oxygen in your blood will remain the same but your ability to transfer oxygen to the cells dramatically reduces. EWOT raises your arterial pressure back to more youthful levels.

EWOT is gaining popularity and while there are limited studies it's reported to have a positive benefit on athletic performance and preventing cancers and other chronic diseases. A company based in the USA has now taken EWOT to the next level by switching between an oxygen-rich and oxygen-reduced air environment ⓡ. This encourages maximum blood flow and oxygenation.

Ozone therapy

Ozone (O3) gas was discovered in the 1840s and has been studied for the past 150 years. Ozone is a toxic and colourless gas made up of just three oxygen atoms. You've probably come across ozone before in relation to the 'hole in the ozone layer' because it's a gas that protects the Earth from ultraviolet radiation.

Ozone therapy is used in medicine to treat wounds by disinfecting the area, improving the body's ability to use oxygen and activating the immune system. This isn't something for you to try at home because you need to work with a specialist. It is used in a medical context to treat a wide range of conditions including infected wounds, cancer, AIDS and macular degeneration.

A 2017 study[3] reviewed studies covering twenty-seven years and concluded that:

'O3 therapy can alter the natural history of several diseases and disorders, with potentially many more yet untested.'

Hyperbaric

Hyperbaric (HBOT) oxygen chambers are best known as a treatment for scuba divers with decompression illness, but most people don't know that it can be used for a wide range of conditions, is excellent for overall wellness, and enhances the body's natural ability to heal.

HBOT is recommended for healing wounds that aren't healing (burns and abscesses) as well as severe conditions. It's become especially popular with multiple sclerosis (MS) treatment, and a lot of the MS centres in the UK now have hyperbaric chambers.

HBOT involves breathing pure oxygen at three times the normal atmospheric pressure which enables the lungs to gather more oxygen. This oxygen is then carried throughout your body to help fight bacteria and stimulate the release of stem cells and growth factors.

HBOT either takes place in a unit designed for one person or in a room designed to accommodate several people. HBOT usually lasts around two hours, and multiple sessions are required. The number of sessions is mainly dependent on the condition being treated.

HBOT is providing an effective procedure for a wide range of chronic conditions, but it appears to be very individual and larger studies are showing conflicting information. More research is needed to prove the efficacy of HBOT, and it may be that it's more effective when combined with other interventions such as a ketogenic diet.[4] Although, the current studies are inconclusive, it's not stopping professional sports teams in the NFL and English Premiership Football from investing in hyperbaric oxygen chambers.

Summary

Breathing calmly is essential to deliver the right amount of oxygen to your lungs and mitochondria while retaining enough carbon dioxide to stop your arteries from contracting. The best way to achieve this is to breathe through your nose rather than your mouth and the breathing techniques that I outlined are an effective way to help you in the moment and are a great antidote to stress. The most important breathing exercise is associated with Heart Rate Variability Training and this will have a huge impact on your ability to manage stress and emotions. Finally, EWOT, ozone therapy and hyperbaric chambers are highly effective therapies that enable you to use and absorb oxygen more effectively.

Your actions:

∞ Concentrate on breathing slow and deep, through your nose. Bring your awareness to this part of your body a few times each day. Notice if you are breathing through your nose or your mouth?

∞ Try nasal breathing and other techniques to optimise your oxygen levels

∞ Purchase an HRV Training Device and practice this daily to help you manage your response to stress and build resilience

∞ Perform your own research into oxygen therapies and identify providers in your local area

Part 3 of this book brings all the actions together in an easy-to-follow checklist.

References

1   Buteyko, K. P. (n.d.). Practical elements. Retrieved from www.buteyko.com/practical/elements/index_elements.html

2   Kim, H. G., Cheon, E. J., Bai, D. S., Lee, Y. H., & Koo, B. H. (2018). Stress and Heart Rate Variability: A Meta-Analysis and Review of the Literature. *Psychiatry investigation*, 15(3), 235–245. PMID: 29486547 – DOI: 10.30773/PI.2017.08.17

3   Smith, N. L., Wilson, A. L., Gandhi, J., Vatsia, S., & Khan, S. A. (2017). Ozone therapy: an overview of pharmacodynamics, current research, and clinical utility. Medical gas research, 7(3), 212–219. PMID: 29152215 – DOI: 10.4103/2045-9912.215752

4   Poff, A. M., Ari, C., Seyfried, T. N., & D'Agostino, D. P. (2013). The ketogenic diet and hyperbaric oxygen therapy prolong survival in mice with systemic metastatic cancer. *PloS one,* 8(6), e65522. PMID: 23755243 – DOI: 10.1371/JOURNAL.PONE.0065522

CHAPTER TWELVE

GETTING COLD MAKES YOU STRONGER

We have become alienated from nature. However, the cold is capable of bringing us back to what we once had lost.

WIM HOF

In this chapter, you will discover:

- ∞ The benefits of cold thermogenesis and why it's important

- ∞ How to get started with cold showers

- ∞ How to take cold showers to the next level with ice baths and cold-water swimming

- ∞ What whole body cryotherapy is and its benefits

Remember to look out for the recommended resources symbol **Ⓡ**.

Do you love the cold?

You love the cold, don't you?

If your answer is YES, then you're in the right place, and if it's NO, then please hear me out because the health and performance benefits are worth your time reading this chapter.

We are very fortunate these days to be able to keep warm with warm clothes, a warm house and a warm car, but we've lost the feeling of being cold and genuinely how amazing you can feel when you get cold. It's not always been this way and humans for thousands of years had to live in an environment where there was extreme cold. Many civilisations actively sought out cold exposure:

∞ The ancient Romans would plunge into frigidarium baths.

∞ The Nordics would crack open the ice on a lake to go swimming in winter.

∞ In the 18th century, Dr Hahn's book *On the Healing Virtues of Cold Water, Inwardly and Outwardly Applied* was published in Germany. Interest reached a peak in the Victorian era, and cold baths were frequently prescribed for all manner of complaints from bruises to hysteria.

Even in modern times, the Finnish know something that most of the world does not. Winter swimming (or ice hole/ pool swimming) is a traditional Finnish outdoor activity.

Wim Hof, a Dutch daredevil, holds twenty-six world records including one for the longest ice bath:

∞ In 2009, he completed a full marathon above the Arctic Circle in Finland, in temperatures of –20°C, dressed in nothing but shorts

∞ In 2009, he reached the top of Mount Kilimanjaro within two days wearing only his shorts

∞ In 2011 he broke his own world record for staying immersed in ice for one hour and fifty-two-minutes

∞ He climbed 22,000 feet up Mount Everest wearing only his shorts and shoes and had to stop due to a foot injury

Wim Hof can withstand such extreme temperatures through controlling his breathing and practising his Wim Hof Method. He has been the focus for much scientific research because his feats have been deemed scientifically impossible. In 2014 a study into the Wim Hof Method concluded that:

'through practicing techniques learned in a short-term training program, the sympathetic nervous system and immune system can indeed be voluntarily influenced'.[1]

MYTH: Getting cold makes you sick.

TRUTH: A cold or flu is associated with cold weather, and therefore many people assume that it's the cold weather that gives you a cold. This is certainly what my mother used to shout at me: 'Put your coat on, or you'll catch your death.' Colds and cases of flu are caused by viruses that just so happen to be more active during the cooler or colder months. For example, the common cold replicates much better when the nose is at 33° to 35° Celsius compared to the core temperature of 37° Celsius.

Cold exposure is often referred to as cold thermogenesis, and the use of ice baths have been used in the world of sports science for the recovery of athletes for a long time, but it's only now becoming clear that they are incredibly useful for energy and performance. Cold thermogenesis is excellent for accelerating healing because when the cold constricts the blood vessels, it reduces blood flow and swelling, and pain and inflammation decrease.

There are many health benefits associated with cold thermogenesis that are backed by scientific studies. These include:

∞ Stimulation of weight loss. Brown adipose tissue (BAT), often referred to as brown fat, is typically found in lean individuals and is rarely found in obese people. A 2013 study[2] concluded that:

   'BAT may serve as a potential target for the treatment and prevention of obesity and other metabolic conditions in humans.'

∞ Reduces sick days. A randomised controlled study in 2016 of 3,018 participants that took a cold shower every day, reported a 29% reduction in sickness days[3]

∞ Increased norepinephrine. A 2008 study[4] showed that cold exposure increased plasma norepinephrine by 200–300%. Norepinephrine is a neurotransmitter found in the brain and is critical for:

   ~ Relief from depression. Higher levels of norepinephrine are also linked with improved mood and people suffering from depression often have low levels of norepinephrine.[5]

   ~ Reducing inflammation. Research[6] shows that norepinephrine plays a role in reducing inflammation.

   ~ Improves cognition. A 2017 review[7] stated that: *'norepinephrine is now recognized as a contributor to various aspects of cognition, including attention, behavioral flexibility, working memory, and long-term mnemonic processes.'*

Taking a cold shower every day

An easy way to get started with cold exposure is to end your daily shower with a one-minute cold shower. You're probably thinking I'm crazy.

Through my process of self-improvement, I've often come across 'the power of a cold shower' and various bloggers and podcasts praising the virtues of freezing yourself every morning, but I thought 'it's not for me'.

CASE STUDY: Having cold showers for thirty days.

The thought of having a cold shower in the morning failed to excite me and quite frankly, it terrified me. I decided to commit to trying a cold shower for one minute every morning for thirty days to see how I felt, and this is what I found:

∞ Day 1 – It felt awful. I stood in the shower and counted one thousand, two thousand and then almost bottled it at thirty thousand, but I finally completed sixty seconds and jumped out of the water. I felt exhilarated, wide awake and focused, and felt a surge of energy as if my blood was rushing through my body.

∞ Day 2 – I was still apprehensive and not sure if the sixty second torture was worth its after-effects. However, I took the plunge and felt the same effects as on day one. At least I knew that it did not happen by luck. I had such a great focus all morning, could it be due to the shower or something else?

∞ Days 3 to 6 – I was still not sure if I liked the cold, but I enjoyed the effects that it had on my mood and concentration first thing in the morning. I decided that it was worth the initial cold shock.

∞ Day 7 – Something strange happened to me on day seven. After about thirty seconds, I could no longer feel the cold water, and it almost felt warm for the last thirty seconds. It's difficult to explain, but it felt like my body temperature was increasing.

∞ Days 8 to 14 – I had begun to enjoy taking a cold shower, including the cold sensation at the start, and loved the feeling of the cold water running down my body and its after-effects as mentioned earlier. This is where something interesting happened to me. In the past twelve months I had been suffering from Raynaud's phenomenon, where my fingers go white when I get too cold. This almost went away and instead, when I felt cold there was a surge of blood to my fingers rather than them turning white. It was as if my circulation had dramatically improved.

∞ Days 15 to 30 – This had now become something that I could not live without, and it occupied a place in my morning routine. I was experiencing its benefits every day, and if you can survive the initial seven days, it's a habit worth developing.

What do you have to lose by trying it? Why not commit to having the last one minute of your shower with cold water every morning for seven days?

If the cold shower is too much for you to start with, then try splashing cold water over your face a few times in the morning and then build up to the cold shower slowly. Alternatively, you can start with a cool shower and each day turn it down gradually. Some people find it beneficial to rub their body rigorously when having a cold shower and that helps them deal with the shock of the cold.

If you find the cold showers to be easy, then try upping the duration to two or three minutes or try alternating between twenty seconds of cold water and ten seconds of hot water for ten iterations.

Stepping it up

Before you advance any further with cold thermogenesis and move on from cold showers, please make sure you are comfortable with being cold and if you have any medical conditions, please remember to check in with your Functional Medical Practitioner first.

Ice baths

Ice baths take the cold shower up several notches, so please be careful when performing an ice bath because if it's too cold, you could give yourself severe burns. You should aim to have the ice bath at around 15°C or 60°F, and the best way to achieve this is to buy bags of ice and add them to a bathtub of water. Lower yourself into the bath and lie down, submerging your body for twenty minutes. This temperature will induce a state of mild cold thermogenesis.

It's best to build yourself up slowly so start with a higher temperature and shorter durations and over time increase the time and decrease the temperature. Don't go too cold because you don't want to have ice burns.

> **CASE STUDY: Tony Robbins and Plunge Pools.**
> Tony Robbins has for many years started his day by jumping into a deep and cold plunge pool (57°F). The exception is where he swims in a river next to his place in Sun Valley, Idaho. Tony talks about the fact that he doesn't enjoy the thought of jumping into the cold water, but it acts as an effective way to tell your mind 'when I say go, we go'.
>
> Tony has since upgraded to cryotherapy and has a chamber in many of his homes.

Swimming in cold water

I'd only suggest this if you are an experienced, strong swimmer and you're aware of the temperature of the water. Strong currents and cramps because of the cold water don't work well together. Always stay safe.

> **CASE STUDY:**
>
> One of my clients has for years swum in the cold open water, and he loves the experience and feeling it gives him. When I asked him what the three most significant benefits were, he replied:
>
> ∞ Focus. You must focus, you must prepare, you must mentally, physically and skill-wise be focused. If not, you'll quickly get in trouble.

∞ Dealing with unpredictability. Tide, weather, your energy, other oddities... are all unpredictable. You get used to it.

∞ Deep mental health benefits. It's silent, repetitive, epiphanic, energetic, difficult, tough, reflective and solo.

∞ A huge back and no obesity concerns. You get huge back muscles, and you can eat whatever you like as you will burn it off.

Get outside when it's cold

It doesn't often happen in the UK, but when it snows, it's an excellent time to get cold, take off (most) of your clothes and go and play in the snow for a few minutes. My son and I did this last year when it had snowed. We ran outside and did snow angels in the snow for forty-five seconds and then had a snowball fight. It was great fun.

If you don't fancy playing in the snow, on a cold day you could go for a walk with just a few layers and embrace the cold weather.

Whole body cryotherapy

Whole body cryotherapy (WBC), invented in Japan in the 1970s, uses a specialised human-sized chamber and liquid nitrogen to induce extreme cold in temperatures of $-110°C$ $(-166°F)$. Fortunately, you only need to spend two or three minutes in the WBC chamber, which is the equivalent of one hour in an ice bath ®.

Cryotherapy works by activating your skin's cold receptors, which then send a message to your brain to constrict the peripheral arteries and send blood directly to your core organs. This results in your blood picking up more nutrients than it would usually pick up. The magic starts when you exit the WBC chamber and return to room temperature because your arteries then dilate, your body systems check-in with what hurts, what needs repair and where the inflammation is. It then sends highly oxidised and nutrient-rich blood to the part of your body where you need it most.

The advantages to cryotherapy over ice baths are:

∞ Reduced time: two to three minutes versus thirty to sixty minutes

∞ The cold is more comfortable than an ice bath

∞ You get to stay dry

∞ The tissues do not freeze, and muscles do not lose capacity, so that athletes can get back to training immediately after a treatment

The downside is that they can be an expensive option for regular use, so I would recommend you use cryotherapy when you have an injury, pain or significant inflammation or a specific condition that you are looking to treat. A 2017 review[8] of the latest cryotherapy literature concluded that:

'the majority of evidence supports effectiveness of WBC in relieving symptomatology of the whole set of inflammatory conditions that could affect an athlete'.

Cryotherapy has for many years been used in professional sports and is now being used by many NFL, English Premiership

Football teams and professional boxers. It's been reported that many of the world's top performers now use cryotherapy to improve their energy and performance.

Summary

The modern world has lost touch with what it means to get cold, and most people have lost the benefits that come with it through a process called cold thermogenesis. It's best to start with a warm shower each morning and at the end have a one-minute cold shower. When you get more comfortable with being cold, you can experiment with an ice bath, taking a walk in the cold or swimming in cold water. If you have a specific condition that you are looking to manage or are concerned about reducing inflammation, then look for a WBC in your area.

Your actions:

- ∞ Commit to having a cold shower at the end of your hot shower for one minute every day for thirty days

- ∞ Once you are comfortable with cold showers try alternating hot and cold

- ∞ Take an ice bath, start slowly and build up the duration and decrease the temperature

- ∞ Experience cryotherapy by checking out a WBC facility or spa in your nearest city

Part 3 of this book brings all the actions together in an easy-to-follow checklist.

References

1   Kox, M., van Eijk, L. T., Zwaag, J., van den Wildenberg, J., Sweep, F. C., van der Hoeven, J. G., & Pickkers, P. (2014). Voluntary activation of the sympathetic nervous system and attenuation of the innate immune response in humans. *Proceedings of the National Academy of Sciences*, 111(20), 7379–84. PMID: 24799686 – DOI: 10.1073/PNAS.1322174111

2   Mund, R. A., & Frishman, W. H. (2013). Brown adipose tissue thermogenesis: -3-adrenoreceptors as a potential target for the treatment of obesity in humans. *Cardiology in review*, 21(6), 265–269. PMID: 23707990 – DOI: 10.1097/CRD.0B013E31829CABFF

3   Buijze, G. A., Sierevelt, I. N., van der Heijden, B. C., Dijkgraaf, M. G., & Frings-Dresen, M. H. (2016). The effect of cold showering on health and work: A randomized controlled trial. *PloS one*, 11(9), e0161749. PMID: 27631616 – DOI: 10.1371/JOURNAL.PONE.0161749

4   Leppäluoto, J., Westerlund, T., Huttunen, P., Oksa, J., Smolander, J., Dugué, B., & Mikkelsson, M. (2008). Effects of long-term whole-body cold exposures on plasma concentrations of ACTH, beta-endorphin, cortisol, catecholamines and cytokines in healthy females. *Scandinavian Journal of Clinical and Laboratory Investigation*, 68(2), 145–153. PMID: 18382932 – DOI: 10.1080/00365510701516350

5   Moret, C., & Briley, M. (2011). The importance of norepinephrine in depression. *Neuropsychiatric disease and treatment*, 7(Suppl 1), 9–13. PMID: 21750623 – DOI: 10.2147/NDT.S19619

6   Yan Liu, X. X. R., Shi, H., Qiu, Y. H., & Peng, Y. P. (2018). Norepinephrine Inhibits Th17 Cells via -2-Adrenergic Receptor (-2-AR) Signaling in a Mouse Model of Rheumatoid Arthritis. *Medical science monitor: international medical journal of experimental and clinical research*, 24, 1196–1204. PMID: 29485127 – DOI: 10.12659/MSM.906184

7   Borodovitsyna, O., Flamini, M., & Chandler, D. (2017). Noradrenergic modulation of cognition in health and disease. *Neural plasticity*, 2017, 6031478. PMID: 28596922 – DOI: 10.1155/2017/6031478

8   Lombardi, G., Ziemann, E., & Banfi, G. (2017). Whole-Body Cryotherapy in Athletes: From Therapy to Stimulation. An Updated Review of the Literature. Frontiers in physiology, 8, 258. PMID: 28512432 – DOI: 10.3389/FPHYS.2017.00258

CHAPTER THIRTEEN

SUPPLEMENTS ARE THE LAST MILE

The supplement industry is the biggest
threat to the pharmaceutical industry.

STEVEN MAGEE

In this chapter you will discover:

∞ Why supplementation isn't where you should start

∞ Why timing and cycling is important

∞ Which supplements are essential for most people

∞ Why intravenous supplements are gaining in popularity

∞ What nootropics and smart drugs are, including my personal experiences of them

Remember to look out for the recommended resources symbol **®**.

The last mile

The supplement industry is a multi-billion-pound industry with an impressive marketing machine, and it's becoming increasingly difficult for you to truly understand what you should and shouldn't be supplementing with. Supplements are often seen as a quick fix for specific ailments, and you are sold the mindset that if you take a multivitamin each day, then you will be healthy. A heavy focus on supplementation should be the 'last mile' of your peak performance journey.

There are many ways to take supplements which include intravenously, topically (on your skin) and up your bottom. I've tried all three, and each is effective. For example, magnesium, iodine and vitamin C work effectively as topical applications, and glutathione is effective as part of a coffee enema. I bet you're thinking 'yuck'.

It is better to meet most of your nutritional needs (vitamins, minerals and amino acids) through your food. Eating a varied and healthy diet which is rich in vegetables should meet most of your dietary requirements. You should focus on your diet, realise the benefits and then target your supplementation to plug specific gaps.

Supplementation is unique to each person because we are all biologically different and have different needs, so taking a broad-brush approach doesn't work. The supplements must be tailored to the individual based on their key biomarkers. It's for this reason that I don't share the supplements that I take daily because while it's right for me, it may not be right for you. I recommend testing to understand what you are deficient in and then selecting your supplementation accordingly.

CASE STUDY: Vitamin B12 deficiency.
When my tests came back, my B12 was 285ng/mL with the normal range being 200–900, so I was on the lower side. The doctor said I was 'within range', but I wasn't happy with the result, so I carried on digging and found that a result between 150 and 400ng/mL is considered borderline and should be evaluated further.

I decided to dig further into my B12 supplementation and based on my genetic profile my body responds best to hydroxocobalamin B12 and not methylcobalamin B12. I started taking oral hydroxocobalamin B12 ⓡ and then switched to intravenous hydroxocobalamin B12, which is far more effective. The things I learned from this:

∞ I may have been feeling OK, but I wasn't performing to the best of my ability

∞ I always need to know my baseline, so I can tell if I need to supplement

∞ There is a difference between the normal range and optimal range

∞ There are different forms of the same supplement, which one is right?

∞ When taking a supplement, sometimes you need to take another one at the same time, ie folate and vitamin B12 together.

The essentials

You are unique, so I don't recommend that you follow my supplementation protocol. However, there are a handful of supplements that everybody should consider taking:

∞ Vitamin D and vitamin K ® (5,000iu in the morning) – in the winter people don't produce enough vitamin D, and therefore you should consider supplementation. Vitamin K works synergistically with vitamin D.

∞ Vitamin C ® (1,000mg in the morning and evening). The recommended dose for vitamin C is very low and when I feel a cold coming on, I will take 3–4 grams of vitamin C per day.

∞ Krill oil ® (2,000mg in the evening) is an excellent source of omega-3 fatty acids.

∞ Magnesium ® (400–500mg in the evening). Most people are deficient in magnesium because it has been depleted from the soil due to over farming. Magnesium-rich foods such as spinach, chard, cabbage and kale no longer contain enough magnesium.

The quality ® of your supplements does matter, and it can start to become very expensive, so you want to ensure that what you're taking is the correct dosage and that it is high-quality so that your body absorbs it.

Timing and cycling your supplements

It's essential to ensure that the time of day is right and whether to take them with or without food. This doesn't mean the supplement won't work but they are more effective based on time of day and whether they are consumed with food.

MYTH: I only need to take a multivitamin each day.

TRUTH: The majority of multivitamins are of poor quality and don't have the correct balance of vitamins and minerals to meet your unique needs. They will often have too little of one vitamin and too much of another. You are also not taking your vitamins at the right time of day to maximise its bio-availability. I challenge you to take any of the fancy well-marketed multivitamins and throw them in the bin.

When you take supplements over an extended period, their efficacy drops significantly, and they don't have the same impact. It's therefore essential that you cycle your supplements to ensure that your body isn't building up a tolerance to the supplements and that you aren't suppressing your body's own natural ability to make it.

I cycle off my supplements:

∞ On a Saturday and Sunday

∞ One week per quarter

∞ When on holiday

Intravenous (IV) vitamins

There is something that I do want to share with you, and that's my experience with intravenous vitamins, which I've now experienced in California and in London. I now take many supplements intravenously because they are more bio-available. It's not something you can do at home, so check out a specialist ® in your area.

> **CASE STUDY:**
> I spoke with a couple of my clients who were suffering from a heavy cold and the start of man flu. I recommended to them to try IV based on my experience in California, so they both went off to London for a Myers Cocktail with glutathione. Both reported back that they felt 100% better within 24 hours.

Nootropics, the smart drugs that work

Nootropics, also known as 'smart drugs', are compounds that enhance your natural memory, neurology, cognition and intelligence. Nootropics can be used for a wide variety of reasons, including increased mental focus, improved memory, anti-ageing, and to improve symptoms of depression. Before you decide to try any nootropics, please consult with a Functional Medical Practitioner.

This is a subject that draws a great deal of interest from many people because it's taboo and gives the impression of a quick fix. Pop a pill and everything will be fixed, and you'll have super-powers. The use of nootropics to create an altered state has skyrocketed in the past few years and a survey conducted by Oxford Universities Newspaper, *The Tab,*[1] showed that 26% of students had tried a nootropic called Modafinil to help increase attention, focus and their ability to learn. It has also been widely reported that the use of nootropics is on the rise in Silicon Valley and for similar reasons micro-dosing LSD (one-fifteenth of a tab) ⓡ is being used to induce a state of focus and creativity. It's generated such interest that in September 2018, the Berkley Foundation and Imperial College London launched the first ever placebo-controlled trial ⓡ of LSD micro-dosing.[2]

Please don't pop a pill because your friend said it was a good idea. Like all things, when something is new, start slowly and build up over time.

Some common nootropics fall into a grey zone from a legal perspective, which means they are not illegal to consume, but it's illegal to purchase them in some geographies. Please do check the legislation in your country, ensure you use a reputable company and please don't break the law.

One of the exciting things about supplementation and nootropics is that what works for me may not work for you and it's not black or white but a sliding scale. I have clients who feel a profound effect on their energy levels when taking a specific nootropic and others feel no difference. The trick is to find out what works for you and to keep an open mind.

I can quite honestly say that I've never smoked a cigarette or taken illegal drugs in my life. Experimenting with nootropics is something that I don't take lightly. There are many nootropics on the market, the ones that I've written about in this chapter are those that I have direct experience with.

Modafinil

Modafinil is probably one of the most popular, especially with students and executives. Modafinil is illegal to purchase in many countries, but it's not illegal to take; therefore, it falls into the 'grey market' category. A 2017 article in the UK newspaper 'The Independent' states that the Cambridge Professor of Clinical Neuropsychology and global expert on cognitive-enhancing drugs, Dr Barbara Sahakian, argues that licensing study drugs to students might be a good idea.[3]

What is it that makes this nootropic so popular? Modafinil increases dopamine release which improves focus, problem-solving, mood and wakefulness. It's not a stimulant that will distract you, it's not addictive, but it may give you a crazy amount of focus.

If you take Modafinil, it needs to be in the morning because it has a half-life of fifteen hours, so it will keep you awake at night if you don't take it first thing in the morning, ie at 7am. Also, be mindful of the fact that Modafinil does not work for everybody and some people are non-responders based on their genetic profile.

I take Modafinil occasionally, and when I do, I achieve a crazy amount of focus, and I can get lost for hours on a project and get so much work done. It has also come in useful when handling jetlag or if I've had a disturbed sleep because it brings me back to my usual mode of performance.

I have experienced a few downsides with Modafinil, which have included a slight level of anxiety, a tendency to be less patient and a lack of empathy. I often feel tired the next day and not as productive, so I've needed to prioritise rest. Modafinil is something that I take only when I need it and when I do, I get strong effects. However, the impact that it has on me the next day makes me feel that it's not something that I would want to take on a regular basis as I want a smooth and consistent level of performance.

CoQ10/ PQQ

Coenzyme Q10 (CoQ10) is an essential nutrient that works as an antioxidant in the body. In its active form, it's called ubiquinol and this needs to be present in cells for your mitochondria to make energy from fat and nutrients. It also defends cells from damage caused by free radicals and increases absorption of other essential nutrients. As you age your ability to produce CoQ10 declines, especially after the age of forty.

Pyrroloquinoline quinone (PQQ), is a compound that helps to form new mitochondria and increases cellular energy production. PQQ brings some significant benefits to your energy levels. It also has antioxidant properties and helps reduce inflammation and boosts brain power.

When taking a CoQ10/PQQ supplement, I feel a quiet surge of energy and my ability to concentrate and focus increases. It's not a jittery surge of energy, but an inner glow that radiates out. I feel it in my brain quickly, it gives me mental clarity, and I feel sharp.

Often PQQ and CoQ10 ® are combined in one supplement. Make sure it is liposomal, ie wrapped in fat to prevent your stomach acid from destroying it.

Aniracetam

Aniracetam ® is a pharmaceutical product developed by Hoffman-La Roche in the 1970s and is part of the racetam family of nootropics, which includes piracetam, oxiracetam and phenylpiracetam.

Aniracetam helps with fluency and working memory, enabling the words to fall out of my head and hit my tongue more easily. It's a subtle nootropic, and many people report that they don't realise the benefits until they stop taking it. There haven't been conclusive human studies that have established that aniracetam is a potent cognitive enhancer, but through my own experiences and others that I know, aniracetam significantly improves my working memory and verbal fluency. When taking aniracetam, I also take choline because it enhances the effect of the aniracetam and mitigates the side effects that some people experience, such as a mild headache.

L-theanine

L-theanine ® is an amino acid and is found in both green and black tea. It elevates levels of gamma-aminobutyric acid (GABA), dopamine and serotonin in the brain and helps with focus and relaxation without drowsiness. Studies on L-theanine have found that it reduces stress and anxiety[4] and improves mental state, alertness and attention.[5] I take L-theanine most days, Monday to Friday, in the evening to relax before I go to bed. I will also occasionally stack L-theanine and Modafinil together to amplify the effects of Modafinil.

Summary

Supplementation is a key to performing well and to help plug any gaps that nutrition can't fill. It's always better to get your vitamins, minerals and amino acids from your diet but it's not always possible. Start with the essentials and park any further investigation into supplements until you have a better idea of your biomarkers. The quality of your supplements is essential so that you absorb them, and you do get what you pay for with supplements.

I mean it when I say exercise caution when experimenting with any supplements or nootropics. Nootropics are incredibly powerful; you can get some significant benefits from taking them, and they will provide a massive boost to your performance exactly when you need it.

Your actions:

∞ Throw away your multivitamins

∞ Purchase the essential supplements that I've listed ®

∞ Use your biomarker testing to target future supplementation (Chapter 5)

∞ Find a credible provider in your area where you can try intravenous supplements

∞ Do your own research on nootropics and ask the experiences of others

∞ Source your nootropics from a legal and reputable company, start slow and see what works for you

Part 3 of this book brings all the actions together in an easy-to-follow checklist.

References

1   Fitzsimons, S., & McDonald, M. (2015, March 31). One in five students
    have used modafinil: Study drug survey results. Retrieved from
    https://thetab.com/2014/05/08/1-in-5-students-have-used-modafinil-study-
    drug-survey-results-14102

2   LSD Microdosing (2018, September 17). Retrieved from
    https://beckleyfoundation.org/microdosing-lsd/

3   Diver, T. (2017, June 24). Let students use drugs to improve their grades,
    says Cambridge scientist. Retrieved from www.independent.co.uk/student/
    news/let-students-use-study-drugs-modafinil-narcotics-sell-at-boots-top-
    cambridge-scientist-barbara-a7806111.html

4   White, D. J., de Klerk, S., Woods, W., Gondalia, S., Noonan, C., & Scholey, A. B.
    (2016). Anti-stress, behavioural and magnetoencephalography effects of
    an l-theanine-based nutrient drink: a randomised, double-blind, placebo-
    controlled, crossover trial. *Nutrients*, 8(1), 53. PMID: 26797633 – DOI:
    10.3390/NU8010053

5   Nobre, A. C., Rao, A., & Owen, G. N. (2008). L-theanine, a natural
    constituent in tea, and its effect on mental state. *Asia Pacific journal of
    clinical nutrition*, 17(S1), 167–168. PMID: 18296328 – DOI: 10.3390/
    NU8010053

CHAPTER FOURTEEN

HACK YOUR BRAIN

We need to understand how our minds
work so we can work our minds better.

JIM KWIK

In this chapter you will discover:

- ∞ Why so many highly successful people meditate and why you should give it a try

- ∞ The five different types of brainwaves that you have and the benefits of each

- ∞ The tools and techniques to shift your brainwaves between different states

- ∞ What neuroplasticity is and how you can teach an old dog new tricks

Remember to look out for the recommended resources symbol ®.

Meditation isn't woo

In my twenties and early thirties, there would be no way in the world you would ever get me to meditate. Absolutely no way. Meditation was for hippies and yogis and not for me. It is funny how many people have an unfavourable view of meditation; they imagine somebody sat cross-legged on the top of a hill, next to a monk or a beautiful person. However, most people are either sitting in bed in the morning or on their favourite seat just having a quiet moment.

I love the moment when I introduce the concept of meditation to a client. I see their facial expressions change, and they start to shift around uncomfortably in their chair. When I ask them if they would like to 'try meditation', they never say 'no', it's nearly always a cautious 'yes'. Most of the time, in the next session, they explain how they really enjoyed the experience of meditation and how it has positively impacted their mood that day.

CASE STUDY:

Simon is a busy technology professional with a demanding job and balancing the usual demands of work, family, community and friends. He was finding that he was getting frustrated with his children, especially his son. Simon started meditation early on in our coaching, and he started to feel the benefits almost immediately. Simon highlighted the following three biggest things he has got from a daily meditation practice:

1. I have developed the means to manage the monkey on my shoulder

2. It helps me to maintain a sense of calm and confidence most of the time

3. Meditation is the start of my day and I get a small sense of achievement every time I do it given it's a goal for me to maintain my streak

These studies used Functional Magnetic Resonance Imaging (fMRI) and Electroencephalography (EEG) technologies to explain how meditation works:

∞ A review published in 2015[1] confirmed that meditation has a positive impact on your neurotransmitters, serotonin, gamma-aminobutyric acid (GABA), dopamine and norepinephrine. These neurotransmitters directly regulate your mood, behaviour and anxiety.

∞ A study[2] published in 2016 showed a significant reduction in cortisol levels after twenty-one days of meditation. Higher cortisol levels are an indicator of stress.

∞ Two studies published in 2014 and 2018 found that yoga and meditation significantly raised Dehydroepiandrosterone sulfate (DHEAS)[3], also known as the 'longevity molecule', and Growth Hormone, also known as the 'fountain of youth'.[4]

∞ A study[5] published in 1995 found that running and meditation had similar effects on mood because both activities produce endorphins.

If that isn't enough, in his book *Tools of Titans* ⓡ, Tim Ferriss interviewed billionaires, icons and world-class performers to discover their tactics, routines and habits. More than 80% of the interviewees have some form of daily mindfulness or meditation practice.[6]

MYTH: **You need to have a quiet mind to benefit from meditation.**

TRUTH: When you do start meditation, most people feel their minds should be quiet, serene and peaceful and it couldn't be further from the truth. You will have days when there is a sense of calmness, but on most days your monkey mind will be talking to you:

'What am I having for lunch today?'

'Why am I even bothering to do this, can we just get on with some stuff?'

'I'm really worried about the meeting I have later today.'

'I wonder how my sister is doing?'

Go with the flow. The act of meditation isn't trying to have a calm mind, the exercise of meditation is bringing yourself back to the task once your mind wanders. The more it wanders, the more you bring yourself back to the practice and the more repetitions you do.

There are many different types of meditation, and I have shared some easy places to start ®.

When you have a brainwave

Brainwaves are produced by electrical pulses from your neurons communicating with each other and are detected using EEG sensors which are placed on the scalp. Your brainwaves will change depending on how you are feeling and what you are doing.

The five major brainwaves are divided into bands and are measured in cycles per second called Hertz (Hz). The following table describes each of the brainwaves and specifies tools and techniques to induce a particular state of being which I will discuss later in this chapter.

Brainwave (Frequency Hz)	You experience it when...	How to access it?
Gamma (38 to 42)	Gamma is the fastest of brainwaves and simultaneously processes information rapidly from different areas of the brain. High gamma activity corresponds to a state of peak performance.	Loving-kindness meditation[7]
Beta (12 to 38)	When you are awake managing the world, solving problems, making decisions and focused on cognitive tasks.	Most people are in a beta state, so it's your default way of operating. If you become stressed and anxious then you will enter a high beta state, which shuts down alpha, theta and delta states.
Alpha (8 to 12)	You will be calm, but alert in a state of presence and 'in the moment'. Your body and mind are in synchronicity, and your intuition is strong.	Meditation, binaural beats, neurofeedback, gratitude and Heart Rate Variability Training.
Theta (3 to 8)	When in theta you are in a highly intuitive and imaginary state.	Deep meditation, daydreaming, dream (REM) sleep.
Delta (.5 to 3)	When you are in deep sleep. In this state healing and regeneration are stimulated.	Deep restorative sleep.

You often hear of people talking about being in a 'flow state' or 'in the zone'.

Being in a state of flow is something that many executives and entrepreneurs wish to create on demand as it puts them in the 'zone' and enables them to operate at peak performance. However, reaching a state of peak performance and being in a state of flow is something that many people strive to make happen, yet so many people struggle to create the right conditions for it to occur. The flow is the optimal state of consciousness and typically occurs at the boundary of the alpha and theta state.

Increasing alpha, theta and gamma brainwaves

Some of the techniques to increase alpha, theta and gamma brainwaves have already been covered in Chapter 4 – Sleep Quality Trumps Quantity and Chapter 11 – Flood your Body with Oxygen. As I've already covered these, I am going to focus the remainder of this chapter on the following:

∞ Gratitude

∞ Binaural beats

∞ Handling being triggered

∞ Sensory deprivation

∞ Neurofeedback

Gratitude

A straightforward, free and effective way to increase alpha brainwaves is to express gratitude. Parents are often telling their children that they 'need to be more grateful' but are adults genuinely grateful themselves? We rush from one thing in life to another and rarely take time to be sincerely thankful for the essential elements in our lives.

When people report as feeling grateful, thankful and appreciative in their daily lives, they also feel more loving, forgiving, joyful and enthusiastic.

EXERCISE: Daily gratitude practice.

Daily Gratitude: once per day, sit still with a piece of paper, close your eyes and focus your breathing on the area of your heart, then allow your body to tell you three things that you're genuinely grateful for that day. Really feel them and then write them down on the piece of paper.

When I do this daily, some days I'm grateful for the people I love, and on other days, it's the small things like feeling the wind on my face or the sun on my back.

'The antidote to fear is gratitude. The antidote to anger is gratitude. You can't feel fear or anger while feeling gratitude at the same time.'

Tony Robbins

EXERCISE: Practice gratitude with your family.

Every evening my wife and I sit with our son in bed, and we all ask each other:

'What three things are you grateful for today?'

We go first, and he goes last; he calls it 'doing gratefuls'. He lies in bed, puts his hand on his heart, lowers his breathing and speaks from his heart. The things that he has expressed have amazed us, with responses that we didn't expect from a little boy, and it has brought tears to our eyes.

It's not because he's a budding Zen-like master. He's like any young boy who loves treats, toys and material things. The process of dropping into your heart and expressing gratitude is where the magic happens.

Binaural beats

In the 1800s a Prussian physicist and meteorologist physicist named Heinrich Wilhelm Dove discovered that listening to two different tones of sound in each ear could change the state of mind. For example, if you heard a tone in your right ear of 300Hz and in your left ear of 295Hz, then your brain gets confused and makes up the 5Hz difference. This difference is called a binaural beat.

The binaural beat makes your brain go into a frequency following response and it then produces brainwaves at the same frequency of 5Hz, which is in the theta state.

If you listen to tones with a larger difference, then you will feel alert and active. Whereas if you listen to tones that are closer together you will feel calm or in a meditative state.

There are many providers online that offer paid for and free binaural beats Ⓡ.

Handling being triggered

This is a technique I learned on my Bulletproof® Training and I use it with all my clients.

Whenever you experience thoughts that cause you to have an emotional response, either internally or externally manifesting itself, you have activated the freeze, fight or flight response and the chances are you're reacting in a non-rational way which is either causing you additional stress or stress to those around you. In this state, you are in high beta mode which shuts off alpha and theta.

A straightforward exercise is to accept the emotional response, welcome it, smile at it and then let it dissipate.

I work with a lot of high achievers, who regularly give themselves a hard time for not achieving more; they need to do better, have more money and do a better job. This is what has driven them to achieve success, but it's no longer serving them. It's adding stress to an already stressful lifestyle. This is their inner critic bubbling up, and it's something that I struggled with for years.

Here is a simple technique to manage any emotional response:

> **EXERCISE: Managing triggers.**
>
> ∞ Listen to your body and when you feel you have been triggered, notice where you feel it in your body
>
> ∞ When you feel it bubbling up, first smile and don't resist it or push it away. Smile and welcome it
>
> ∞ Give it a name (say 'Bob') and say to yourself internally, 'that's my Bob, I'm pleased you're here'

This will give time for the rational part of your brain to kick in and help you to move from high beta to low beta. This is particularly effective if then followed by a breathing exercise to move you towards an alpha state.

Sensory deprivation

Developed in the 1950s by Dr John C. Lilly, flotation tanks ® are dark and soundproof pods used for floating in warm magnesium-rich water. The aim of their development was to experiment and explore further with the human consciousness.

There have been a few small scientific studies done on flotation tanks and the mechanisms by which it works are not fully understood due to so many sensory stimuli being altered during floating. A 2018 study[8] examined the antidepressant effect of floating and stated:

'Moreover, participants reported significant reductions in stress, muscle tension, pain, depression and negative affect, accompanied by a significant improvement in mood characterized by increases in serenity, relaxation, happiness and overall well-being.'

Floating is becoming more popular, and it's well established that relaxation is good for you and so is bathing in Epsom salts. Floating attracts people due to the benefits they have experienced, which include:

∞ It helps to manage pain by removing the force generated by gravity, helping your muscles to relax, and relieving pressure and stress.

∞ It increases brain function because it enables your brain to be dominant in alpha and theta brain waves. This is the same state you reach with meditation.

∞ It helps manage stress by activating your parasympathetic nervous system. This results in the release of endorphins and dopamine which help with pain relief and mood enhancement.

∞ It enables magnesium absorption because it contains a high concentration of Epsom salts.

I use flotation tanks to hit the reset button and to spend some time focusing on myself.

Neurofeedback

Neurofeedback ® is an advanced biohack requiring specialised equipment and can be relatively expensive. It involves measuring the brainwaves using sensors to understand the current state of the brain and then to use external stimuli such as sound or light to train your brain. This results in something called neuroplasticity, which is where your brain changes and adapts to create new connections.

MYTH: **You can't teach an old dog new tricks.**

TRUTH: It's been long thought that once you reach adulthood your brain is fixed and you're unable to learn new things. The term 'you can't teach an old dog new tricks' is commonly used by older people, but it's not true. Neuroplasticity is your brain's ability to adapt, create new connections and learn.

Neurofeedback is being used as an alternative treatment and in a 2016 review[9] it was shown to improve ADHD, anxiety, depression, epilepsy, insomnia, drug addiction, schizophrenia, learning disabilities and dyslexia. However, the review did also point out that it can be expensive and take a long time to see the desired results. It's not a short-term fix.

Neurofeedback is quickly gaining traction, and there are centres in Europe and the USA ⓡ where you can have neurofeedback training in week-long retreats. Tony Robbins is quoted on one of their testimonials as saying it's 'one of the most valuable things I've done in my life'.

Summary

You may read this chapter and think that meditation isn't for you, but what have you got to lose by trying it and seeing if it benefits you in some way? It could have a significant impact on your life.

There are five key brainwaves: gamma, beta, alpha, theta and delta, and depending on which of these brainwaves are dominant at any one time, these will alter your state of being. You can train your brain to put yourself into certain states through a combination of technology and techniques. Practising gratitude, meditation and handling triggers are zero cost and things that you can start today. Binaural Beats and HRV Training require a small investment, but the rewards are worth your investment. Neurofeedback is a powerful technology that is rapidly gaining traction and is likely to become more mainstream over the next five years.

Your actions:

∞ Download a meditation app to your smartphone and start to meditate for ten minutes each day, increasing to twenty minutes ®

∞ Take a moment in your day to stop, slow down and reflect what 'state' you've been in in the past thirty minutes and which of the brainwaves you think have been dominant

∞ Take time each day to practice gratitude, especially if you have children

- ∞ Do the exercise on handling triggers and start by noticing when you are triggered and take yourself out of that state

- ∞ Purchase binaural beats and experiment with them when you are doing different tasks and see how you feel ®

- ∞ Research if there are any flotation tanks in your area and give it a go, it's a great experience ®

- ∞ Check out if there are any Neurofeedback providers ® in your area, speak to them and try it out for a few sessions

Part 3 of this book brings all the actions together in an easy-to-follow checklist.

References

1   Krishnakumar, D., Hamblin, M. R., & Lakshmanan, S. (2015). Meditation and yoga can modulate brain mechanisms that affect behavior and anxiety - A modern scientific perspective. *Ancient science*, 2(1), 13–19. PMID: 26929928 – DOI: 10.14259/AS.V2I1.171

2   Bansal, A., Mittal, A., & Seth, V. (2016). Osho Dynamic Meditation's Effect on Serum Cortisol Level. *Journal of clinical and diagnostic research: JCDR*, 10(11), CC05-CC08. PMID: 28050359 – DOI: 10.7860/JCDR/2016/23492.8827

3   Kumar, K., Kumar, D., Singh, V., & Pandey, P. T. (2018). Role of yoga and meditation on serum DHEAS level in first year medical students. *International Journal of Research in Medical Sciences*, 6(6). DOI: 10.18203/2320-6012.IJRMS20182280

4   Chatterjee, S., & Mondal, S. (2014). Effect of regular yogic training on growth hormone and dehydroepiandrosterone sulfate as an endocrine marker of aging. *Evidence-Based Complementary and Alternative Medicine: eCAM*, 2014, 240581. PMID: 24899906 – DOI: 10.1155/2014/240581

5   Harte, J. L., Eifert, G. H., & Smith, R. (1995). The effects of running and meditation on beta-endorphin, corticotropin-releasing hormone and cortisol in plasma, and on mood. *Biological Psychology*, 40(3), 251–265. PMID: 7669835 – DOI: 10.1016/0301-0511(95)05118-T

6 Ferriss, T. (2016, October 25). Tools of Titans – Sample Chapter and a Taste of Things to Come, What do they have in common. Retrieved from https://tim.blog/2016/10/25/tools-of-titans/

7 Lutz, A., Greischar, L. L., Rawlings, N. B., Ricard, M., & Davidson, R. J. (2004). Long-term meditators self-induce high-amplitude gamma synchrony during mental practice. *Proceedings of the national Academy of Sciences*, 101(46), 16369–16373. PMID: 15534199 – DOI: 10.1073/PNAS.0407401101

8 Feinstein, J. S., Khalsa, S. S., Yeh, H. W., Wohlrab, C., Simmons, W. K., Stein, M. B., & Paulus, M. P. (2018). Examining the short-term anxiolytic and antidepressant effect of Floatation-REST. PloS one, 13(2), e0190292. PMID: 29394251 – DOI: 10.1371/JOURNAL.PONE.0190292

9 Marzbani, H., Marateb, H. R., & Mansourian, M. (2016). Neurofeedback: a comprehensive review on system design, methodology and clinical applications. *Basic and clinical neuroscience*, 7(2), 143–58. PMID:27303609 – DOI: 10.15412/J.BCN.03070208

BRINGING IT ALL TOGETHER

Part 2 of this book contains so much useful information, actions, next steps and links to resources. Part 3 brings all of this together into actionable checklists. I'm often asked the question: 'How do I build these strategies into my daily life, so they become a habit?' So, I have created a chapter to help answer this question. Finally, I have included some more detailed case studies from some of my clients so that you can see how they have implemented the strategies from Part 2.

CHAPTER FIFTEEN

HOW TO MAKE THE STRATEGIES A HABIT

> *Excellence is an art won by training and habituation. We do not act rightly because we have virtue or excellence, but we rather have those because we have acted rightly. We are what we repeatedly do. Excellence then is not an act but a habit.*
>
> **ARISTOTLE**

I often find that people are looking for the magic pill, the smart cut to the hack that gives them instant benefit. There are of course tools, techniques, hacks and smart cuts that can give you an immediate boost, but solid habits and routines can't be beaten. You can have all the hacks in the world, but if you're going to make a step change in your life, then you need to build a series of routines which you perform automatically as part of your everyday life.

In this chapter, you will discover how to create a habit that sticks and how you can sequence habits together to form a routine that over time will become as natural as brushing your teeth or charging your phone before bed. You will also learn how to replace bad habits with good habits to create powerful changes.

Remember to look out for the recommended resources symbol ⓡ.

Habits and routines

I like to define a habit as something that you do on a consistent and regular basis to the point where it's as common as taking a shower each morning or taking a glass of water to bed at night. When you build out habits and make them habitual, it has a powerful impact on your life, nudging you in the right direction and setting you up for success. Through the power of neuroplasticity (Chapter 14 – Hack your brain), your mind develops new neuropathways that enable these habits to stick.

I define a routine as stringing many habits together. Routines are more potent than habits because you're able to string a series of habits together and the sum of the whole is much more powerful than the sum of the parts.

You can create many different types of rituals, including:

- ∞ Morning routine – set up your day for success

- ∞ Prepare for sleep routine – prime the next morning and ensure good sleep hygiene

- ∞ Get home from work routine – leave your work on the doorstep and embrace your family time

- ∞ Commute on train routine – prepare for the working day ahead

- ∞ Exercise routine – prime your exercise routine to make sure it happens

∞ End of work routine – wrap up work and plan the next day

∞ Weekly review – review the previous week and set up the next week's priorities

Routines should evolve, and it's best to keep them to a small number of habits and then grow them over time because rushing to create a routine with a long string of habits is much more likely to fail.

Your routines should become the non-negotiable anchors in your life that are there for you; nothing should come before them. Your routines shouldn't be overly complicated or lengthy in duration, and they must serve you, and if they don't, they aren't the right ones.

Many people have asked me where I found the time to write this book given that I already seemed to have a lot going on in my life. The answer is, make it a habit and think about how to use your time effectively.

How to design a routine

To design your routine, there are seven simple steps that you must complete.

1. Start slowly and build incrementally: If you try and do everything at once you are likely to fail. Start with no more than two new things you want to build into your routine and when they become habitual, add more.

2. Understand your why? There are times when you want to avoid the routine and hit the snooze button,

but if you understand why you're doing this and why it's important to you, then you are more likely to act.

3. Write it down: By having a written implementation plan, step by step, then you are three times more likely to perform the routine.

4. Prime: Make things easy on yourself and get things ready in advance. For example, ensure everything is prepared the night before, which includes the clothes that you will wear, bag packed, electronics charged, headphones in the home office and Bulletproof® Coffee ingredients ready in the kitchen.

5. Time your routine: Understand how long your routine takes you and allow enough time.

6. Stay accountable: Work with an accountability partner to help keep you on track.

7. Track it: Don't break the chain. Track the completion of your habits, keep a log and track your streak rate.

Morning routines

Having a solid morning routine is one of the best routines to develop because setting yourself up for success each day is one of the most important things you can do, and designing a morning routine that works is a compelling exercise. Tony Robbins refers to this as priming your day. You're putting yourself in the right physical, emotional and mental state to own your day and make it a success. You can see my morning routine ® in *Resources*.

There are times when I've not done my morning routine, and I feel like my day hasn't gone quite as well. This may well be psychological, but there is more to it than that.

An important point to note with a morning routine is that it needs to tie in with your evening routine, to save time and make the morning as friction-free as possible. For example, the night before I prepare my coffee ingredients, headphones for meditation and clothes for the next day.

The biggest problem for your morning routine is going to be the time that you go to bed, so you must have a set time for bed each night, which you stick to as much as you can. For example, in bed by 10pm and wake at 5.50am.

There will be times where during the weekdays there may be work or social commitments that mean that you need to go to bed later and wake up late, which throws your morning routine into chaos. In these circumstances, shorten your morning routine to the things that you get the most benefit from.

As part of your morning routine, never check social media, the news or email. It will only take one email to throw your day off course.

Replacing bad habits with good habits

We all have some bad habits. The things that you do and, afterwards, you regret doing, but you can't help yourself. There is an element of guilt once you've performed the bad habit, which may be immediate and obvious or comes with pangs of guilt that kick in afterwards.

I classify bad habits as something that you're doing that you don't want to be doing and that get in the way of the things that you do want to do. Here are the top five bad habits that I've noticed with my clients:

∞ Procrastinating and allowing distraction rather than acting

∞ Drinking too much alcohol and self-medicating rather than tackling the cause of their problems

∞ Watching too much Netflix rather than winding down ready for bed

∞ Snacking on sugar rather than a healthy alternative

∞ Working too much rather than focusing on health and spending time with friends and family

How to change the negative habit loop

Firstly, identify the trigger, routine and reward that relates to the habit. For example: snacking on sugar rather than a healthy alternative. In this example, you may be feeling low on energy at 11am (trigger), you walk past the vending machine at work (routine), and you buy a chocolate bar from the vending machine (reward).

Secondly, identify what is causing the trigger? Are there underlying emotions or other habits that are leading to a bad habit? In this example, you may well not be having enough nourishment at breakfast. Having a healthy breakfast may eliminate or reduce this trigger.

Thirdly, accepting that a trigger exists, what different routine can you put in place? For example: having healthy snacks at hand that are low in sugar. Therefore, your routine becomes to go to your office locker and choose a healthy snack and eat it outside in the sunshine. Eating outside has the added benefit of getting you out in the fresh air (reward).

Using this three-step process, which bad habits do you think you can turn into good habits?

When your routine drops

You will find that from time to time your habits and routines will drop off and it's usually due to a change in environment such as travelling with work, holiday, change in working location or visitors to your home. These are temporary interruptions, are part of life, and are not something that you should be concerned about.

Where possible, try and pre-empt this and recognise that you cannot do your full routine and change it accordingly. For example, if you don't have access to a gym while on a business trip then have a backup plan, such as the seven-minute workout, and reduce your morning meditation from twenty minutes to ten minutes.

You will also find that your habits and routines may suddenly drop, and you won't think about them for a few days until you take a moment to step back and realise that you've been super busy. You'll also probably promise yourself to start back on Monday because it's a fresh start to the week, even though it may be a Thursday or Friday. The unfortunate reality is that when you allow your life to take over and you get busy, usually with work, the first thing that happens is that you stop putting yourself first and your habits and routines go out of the window, even though this is the time when you need them the most. Use this as an early warning sign that something isn't right and you're probably under stress.

If you find that your routines stop then:

- ∞ Stop, slow down and reflect. Check in with yourself, what is going on in your life and why have you dropped your routines.

- ∞ Go back and review why the routines are important to you. Connect back in with the more profound reason as to why you do them.

- ∞ Start again tomorrow and not on Monday. When you're in a busy or stressed state, you need your habits and routines more than ever.

There is an old Zen saying: *'You should sit in meditation for twenty minutes a day unless you're too busy. Then you should sit for an hour.'*

Summary

In this chapter, you learned what habits and routines are and how to design your routines, so that you can integrate into your life what you learned in Part 2 – Twelve strategies for limitless energy and peak performance. A good place to start is a morning routine because it sets your day up for success. You also learned how to replace bad habits with good ones, how to track your routines and what to do when your routines drop.

CHAPTER SIXTEEN

ACTIONABLE CHECKLISTS

This chapter contains a series of checklists, which combines all the actions from the chapters in Part 2. There are checklists for:

∞ If you do nothing else, do these

∞ Starting out

∞ Going further

∞ Stepping it up a level

Remember to look out for the recommended resources symbol Ⓡ.

If you do nothing else, do these

Here is a list of five things that are free, you can start immediately, and they will make a significant difference to your performance within one week:

Chapter 3 – Eat what makes you feel great

☐ Take the time after each meal and snack to make a note of how you feel. If you don't feel great, ie low energy, brain fog or bloating, then question what was in the food.

Chapter 7 – Move more and exercise less

☐ Bring High Intensity Interval Training (HIIT) into your exercise regime, both cardio and strength based ®

Chapter 12 – Getting cold makes your stronger

☐ Commit to having a cold shower at the end of your hot shower for one minute every day for thirty days

Chapter 14 – Hack your brain

☐ Download a meditation app ® for your smartphone and start to meditate for ten minutes each day, increasing to twenty minutes

☐ Take time each day to practice gratitude, especially if you have children

Starting out

Chapter 3 – Eat what makes you feel great

☐ Find a local source and purchase: a) grass-fed, grass-finished meat ® b) organic vegetables ® c) wild-caught fish ®

Chapter 4 – Sleep quality trumps quantity

☐ Buy a sleep tracking device and track every day ®

☐ Complete the actions in 'Hacking Sleep' – find out what works for you

☐ Don't drink any caffeine after 2pm

☐ Keep alcohol to a minimum

☐ Keep the room cool

☐ Create a bedtime routine

☐ Watch your exercise at night

☐ Get to bed before 11pm

☐ Write a journal for ten minutes

☐ Put your phone on the other side of the room

Chapter 5 – What gets measured gets managed

☐ Measure and track your activity and the quality of your sleep each night ®

☐ Track your physical biomarkers and set a reminder to review them on a regular basis

☐ Buy a basic blood panel ® or ask your doctor for the tests

Chapter 6 – Burning fat for fuel

☐ Drink Bulletproof® Coffee ® in the morning and see how you feel when the exogenous ketones hit your brain

☐ Check out the Resources and identify the foods higher in omega 3s and build them into your diet ®

Chapter 7 – Move more and exercise less

- ☐ Consider how much you are exercising, are you exercising enough or are you over-exercising? What do you need to change?

- ☐ Move more, find ways to increase the amount of movement you do each day

Chapter 8 – Embracing the magic of light

- ☐ Ask yourself the question, are you getting enough sunshine and what can you do to get more during your day?

- ☐ Where are you exposed to junk light in your life and what can you do to avoid it?

Chapter 9 – Not all water is equal

- ☐ Buy a drinks container to enable you to get more fluids in each day ®

- ☐ Follow the guidelines on how to stay hydrated by anchoring your drinking to specific events in your day

Chapter 10 – Toxins will kill your performance

- ☐ Ensure that in your home you have plenty of ventilation

- ☐ Check all pipework on a regular basis for water leaks. Where you do have a mould problem, have it properly treated, and the root cause addressed.

☐ Ensure there is no visible sign of mould in your food and take note that most of the time mould can be invisible to the human eye

☐ Go through your garden shed, throw away anything that contains glyphosate and use a natural weed killer, such as your hands or a solution of salt and vinegar ®

☐ Eat organic whenever possible – the list of foods being sprayed with glyphosate is proliferating and is too long to list here ®

Chapter 11 – Flood your body with oxygen

☐ Concentrate on breathing slow and deep, through your nose. Bring your awareness to this part of your body a few times each day. Notice: am I breathing through my nose or mouth?

☐ Try the breathing exercises, they do work and are very effective

Chapter 13 – Supplements are the last mile

☐ Throw away your multivitamins

☐ Purchase the essential supplements that I've listed ®

Chapter 14 – Hack your brain

☐ Take a moment in your day to stop, slow down and reflect what 'state' you've been in in the past thirty minutes and which of the brainwaves you think have been dominant

☐ Do the exercise on handling triggers and start by noticing when you are triggered and take yourself out of that state

Going further

Chapter 3 – Eat what makes you feel great

☐ Commit for a month to eliminate the foods in this chapter and see how you feel

☐ Bring more foods into your diet that are high in polyphenols Ⓡ

Chapter 4 – Sleep quality trumps quantity

☐ Complete the exercise to understand how much sleep you need each day, what time you should go to bed and wake up. Experiment with this to find your sweet spot

☐ Complete the actions in 'Hacking sleep'. Find out what works for you

　☐ Drink honey, tea and apple cider vinegar before bed

　☐ Avoid blue lights at night

　☐ Take a magnesium supplement Ⓡ

Chapter 5 – What gets measured gets managed

☐ Measure your Heart Rate Variability Ⓡ to track your stress and recovery levels

☐ Have your gut microbiome tested Ⓡ

Chapter 6 – Burning fat for fuel

☐ Cut back your carbohydrates to 30–50g a day

☐ Eat two meals a day between the hours of 2pm and 8pm

☐ Measure your ketones using a ketone blood monitor Ⓡ

Chapter 7 – Move more and exercise less

☐ Get outside in your bare feet and connect with the earth

Chapter 8 – Embracing the magic of light

☐ Pick up high-quality sunscreen Ⓡ

☐ Purchase blue-blocking glasses Ⓡ

Chapter 9 – Not all water is equal

☐ Do your research on tap water and make an intentional decision

☐ Purchase activated charcoal and glutathione for your next night out Ⓡ

Chapter 10 – Toxins will kill your performance

☐ Minimise your exposure to EMFs by keeping your phone in aeroplane mode when it's in your pocket

☐ Move your Wi-Fi router as far away as possible from where you spend most of the time

☐ Put any wearable devices on aeroplane mode when not required to sync data

☐ Consider taking molecular hydrogen to help mop up any free radicals ®

Chapter 11 – Flood your body with oxygen

☐ Try nasal breathing to optimise your oxygen levels

☐ Purchase an HRV Training Device ® and practice this daily to help you manage your response to stress and build resilience

Chapter 12 – Getting cold makes you stronger

☐ Once you are comfortable with cold showers, try alternating to hot and cold

☐ Take an ice bath, start slowly and build up the duration, and decrease the temperature

Chapter 13 – Supplements are the last mile

☐ Use your biomarker testing to target future supplementation

☐ Do your own research on nootropics and ask the experiences of others

Chapter 14 – Hack your brain

☐ Purchase binaural beats and experiment with them when you are doing different tasks and see how you feel ®

Stepping it up a level

Chapter 3 – Eat what makes you feel great

☐ Grow broccoli seeds at home for sulforaphane ®

Chapter 4 – Sleep quality trumps quantity

☐ When you next take a flight, try out the suggestions to beat jet lag and see what works for you

Chapter 5 – What gets measured gets managed

☐ Purchase a more advanced blood panel ® and a hormone panel ®

☐ Have your DNA sequenced ® and run the results through online diagnostic tools ®

Chapter 6 – Burning fat for fuel

☐ Try a twenty-four hour fast one day when there is nothing suitable to eat

☐ Try a three-day water fast to experience the benefits of keeping deep in ketosis

Chapter 7 – Move more and exercise less

☐ Use a vibration plate at home or at your local gym

Chapter 8 – Embracing the magic of light

- ☐ Purchase an infrared light ®
- ☐ Get screened for Irlen Syndrome ®

Chapter 9 – Not all water is equal

- ☐ Purchase molecular hydrogen tablets ® and take them most days to enjoy the performance and health-span benefits

Chapter 11 – Flood your body with oxygen

- ☐ Perform your own research into oxygen therapy and identify providers in your local area

Chapter 12 – Getting cold makes you stronger

- ☐ Experience cryotherapy by checking out a facility or spa in your nearest city

Chapter 13 – Supplements are the last mile

- ☐ Find a credible provider in your area where you can try intravenous supplements

- ☐ Source your nootropics from a good legal company, start slow and see what works for you

Chapter 14 – Hack your brain

☐ Check out if there are any neurofeedback providers in your area, speak to them and try it out for a few sessions ®

☐ Research if there are any flotation tanks in your area and give it a go, it's a great experience ®

CHAPTER SEVENTEEN

REAL-WORLD CASE STUDIES

Here are four real-world case studies, so you can see how some of my clients have adopted many of the strategies from this book. I have changed their names in the interest of confidentiality.

Matt

You met Matt earlier in the book. He is a Business Director, working with some of the largest investment banks and wealth management firms around the globe.

The situation:

When I first started coaching Matt, he was struggling to focus, and his cognitive performance wasn't where he wanted it to be. He found it difficult to concentrate and was under immense pressure from a very demanding boss. His stress levels were high, and his work/life balance was deteriorating Things weren't going well for Matt, and over a few weeks he had fallen off the rails, was burnt out and was partying hard, which was further impacting his work/life balance. The result was overbearing work stress, and a meltdown at home.

What we did:

Through our coaching sessions, Matt identified what he needed to change but struggled to take the initial first step forward. We spoke about Matt putting himself first, finding his inner calm and being in the best possible headspace to look after his career and his personal life. I love working with clients like Matt because they come with an open mind and are happy to experiment to see what works for them. We worked together on a daily routine to help set each day up for success:

∞ A meditation practice for ten minutes each morning to help calm the mind (Chapter 14 – Hack your brain)

∞ Daily journaling including a gratitude practice to give time for reflection (Chapter 14 – Hack your brain)

∞ A Bulletproof® Coffee to help switch on his brain in the morning to boost his focus (Chapter 6 – Burning fat for fuel)

This simple exercise gave Matt enough of a platform to see clearly and start to address what was going on with him internally, in his workplace and also with his personal life. Matt worked hard to maintain a consistent morning routine and then focused his efforts on:

∞ Listening to his body and eating the foods that made him feel great and avoiding the ones that took away his energy (Chapter 3 – Eat what makes you feel great)

∞ He then stepped this up with a gut microbiome test, so he could understand what foods his microbiome responds best to (Chapter 5 – What gets measured gets managed)

∞ Having bloodwork done to assess his biomarkers – he had low vitamin D and B12 (Chapter 5 – What gets measured gets managed)

∞ Hitting the gym for High-Intensity Interval Training several times per week (Chapter 7 – Move more and exercise less)

∞ Targeting his supplementation to maximise his energy levels, particularly coenzyme Q10 and PQQ in advance of big meetings (Chapter 13 – Supplements are the last mile)

∞ Intravenous vitamins to give his body a much-needed boost (Chapter 13 – Supplements are the last mile)

∞ Taking a cold shower each morning to boost his energy levels (Chapter 12 – Getting cold makes you stronger)

∞ Focusing on improving his quality and not his quantity of sleep (Chapter 4 – Sleep quality trumps quantity)

The result:

Matt immersed himself in the coaching process and quickly realised that each new strategy that he adopted had a compounded effect. Matt started to hit his groove and become emotionally, mentally and physically stronger. He put himself first, and in doing so he was able to rebuild his personal life, and he secured a new role. Matt went on to secure a new position for £100,000 a year more than his last role and is in the process of starting up his own coaching practice in London.

Tom

Tom is an investment banking professional specialising in Electronic Trading risk for a large American Bank.

The situation:

When I first started working with Tom, it wasn't immediately apparent why he wanted coaching because he had a hugely successful career and a lovely family at home in Ireland. Through our sessions, it became evident that although Tom was highly successful, he knew that there was 'more in the tank' and he wanted to find a way to access it. The demands of commuting from Ireland to London were taking its toll and he would often arrive home and have little energy for his wife and two boys. Tom knew there was a greater level to his own personal performance but didn't know how to access it.

What we did:

Being a highly driven person, Tom accelerated through the coaching programme and dived deep into recommended reading and would arrive at our sessions with a real thirst for knowledge. Over a short period, Tom focused on:

- ∞ Intermittent fasting to boost his energy levels and promote autophagy. He then stepped it up to a five-day fast, which he intends on doing each quarter (Chapter 6 – Burning fat for fuel)

- ∞ Cleaning up his diet:

    - ~ Eating what made him feel great and noticing what foods didn't, ie those foods potentially high in mould (Chapter 3 – Eat what makes you feel great)

- ~ After initially moving to a vegan-based diet, he then moved back to a small to moderate amount of high-quality protein (Chapter 3 – Eat what makes you feel great)

- ~ Took a gut microbiome test to target his diet further (Chapter 5 – What gets measured gets managed)

- ∞ Meditation in the gym or at home when things got stressful (Chapter 14 – Hack your brain)

- ∞ Avoiding junk light by wearing blue-blocking glasses at night and in the office (Chapter 8 – Embracing the magic of light)

- ∞ Having bloodwork done to assess his biomarkers, he discovered that he had low vitamin D, and a slightly abnormal liver function (Chapter 5 – What gets measured gets managed)

The result:

Within a couple of weeks Tom's energy levels shot through the roof, and he had more energy than he had ever experienced before. He was able to arrive home in Ireland with energy and spend quality time with his wife and children. In three months he lost seven kilograms in weight and was the lightest he had been since he was twenty-one years old. His work became effortless, and he started to question playing a bigger game in life and what he could do to have more impact on the world.

Paul

Paul is an entrepreneur who co-founded a successful business that helps organisations manage their mergers and acquisitions.

The situation:

Paul like many entrepreneurs worked incredibly hard building a successful business. He found sleep particularly challenging and would often wake up in the early hours of the morning and then struggle to get back to sleep again; especially if there were work issues in play, he would ping wide awake, although his body needed more sleep. Paul also has a pre-determined view on how long he was going to live and felt that the clock was ticking. In addition, Paul had noticed in his network that a small percentage of entrepreneurs appeared to build very demanding businesses and keep their health at peak performance, something he wanted to also achieve. He wanted to live a long and healthy life and wanted to be around to see his daughter growing up. Paul wasn't living a particularly unhealthy lifestyle, but he felt he could be doing a lot more; he just didn't know where to start and what to do.

What we did:

We started by tackling Paul's sleep issues and he started experimenting with the sleep hacks in Chapter 4 – Sleep quality trumps quantity. Paul was tracking his sleep but the device he was using wasn't effective, so he switched to a new device and focused his efforts on ensuring he was getting high-quality deep sleep and that his resting heart rate was low at night. Paul's sleep is much improved; using a device that prioritises sleep quality over physical activity, he can focus on determining what does and doesn't enable him to have a great night's sleep.

Prior to starting a business and starting a family Paul could spend hours exercising or going to the gym. Tackling the limiting beliefs around his health-span required a number of actions that enabled Paul to measure his baseline and feel better, healthier and stronger.

Paul focused his attentions on:

∞ Performing High-Intensity Interval Training (HIIT) twice per week. He performed HIIT at home, which had a dual-benefit of teaching his young daughter about the benefits of exercise in a 'show, not tell' fashion. (Chapter 7 – Move more and exercise less)

∞ Utilising a device to perform meditation while commuting on public transportation. (Chapter 14 – Hack your brain)

∞ Listening to his body and understanding which foods and drinks were impacting him. These were gluten and alcohol. (Chapter 3 – Eat what makes you feel great)

∞ Understanding what some of his baseline bloods were. (Chapter 5 – What gets measured gets managed)

∞ Understanding what his gut microbiome responds best to in terms of foods. (Chapter 5 – What gets measured gets managed)

∞ Taking a small number of targeted supplements. (Chapter 13 – Supplements are the last mile)

The result:

Paul's deeper thoughts on his outlook on life and how long he is likely to live are now dramatically different which, in turn, resulted in more positive and physical activity – further enhancing his physical and mental well-being.

Simon

Simon is an entrepreneur running a start-up which is challenging the traditional recruitment and consultancy models.

The situation:

When I first started coaching with Simon he was at the early stages of creating his business, and as such he was working long hours in the business and on the business at the same time. In addition, he was also writing his book and a demanding business accelerator course. Simon was getting frustrated with himself because he had low energy on the weekends and wasn't present for his family; the weekend was used to recharge for the week ahead. The demands of running a business and not putting himself first also meant that he had put on more weight than he wanted, and he was struggling with brain fog.

What we did:

Simon was hungry for information and he went through periods of time when some of the habits stuck but then tended to drift away when he got busy (Chapter 16 – How to make the strategies a habit). He needed time to let things settle in his mind and when he started to put himself first, he found that several habits started to stick. The things that Simon worked on were:

∞ HIIT in the gym to maximise his workout.
(Chapter 7 – Move more and exercise less)

∞ Introducing time for reflection into his morning
routine to level his mind first thing in the morning.
(Chapter 14 – Hack your brain)

∞ Understanding which foods and drinks were impacting
him and giving him brain fog. (Chapter 3 – Eat what
makes you feel great)

∞ Taking time to get cold each morning with a cold
shower. (Chapter 12 – Getting cold makes you stronger)

The result:

Simon no longer fell into the weekend, using it to recover
and recharge before the next working work. He's ending
the week with energy in the tank despite running a start-up
which is challenging conventional wisdom, and can spend
quality time with his family. He has lost 2.5 stone in weight
and his body fat has dropped from 29% to 12% because
he's prioritised the elements he wanted coaching on. He
is making better decisions for his business and his family
because he is now aware of what takes his energy away.

CONCLUSION

You now understand how your body makes energy through mitochondria and just how important they are, not just to your energy but also to your overall performance and health-span. If your mitochondria are performing well then you are going to have limitless energy, perform better in all parts of your life and increase your chances of achieving a long health-span. You are living at a time where we are understanding in greater detail how we function biologically and what powers us up and knocks us back. Fundamentally, doing everything to support and protect your mitochondria is a great strategy.

There are twelve strategies in Part 2 of this book that will make an incredible difference to your performance. When you start bringing these into your life you will feel the benefits and it's going to give you great results in both your personal and professional life. The key thing is to put yourself first, before your family and work. There is a lot of information in Part 2, so it is something you will want to revisit on a regular basis as you start to build up your habits. This is just the tip of the iceberg in terms of resources and there are many more that I can share with you in the future.

Having all the actions from Part 2 is great but information is useless unless you can embed it into your life. Part 3 provides a series of checklists, so you can start your journey at your pace with guidance on how to build the strategies and actions into your life and how to make more time for them. I've also included some real-life case studies from clients, so you can understand what has worked for them.

If you start on this path you will never look back, you will feel amazing and things will start to click into place around you. It's hard to explain but because you are performing at such a level the decisions you make and the positivity you emit means that the opportunities come to you.

What's next?

If you would like to find out more about my Human Optimisation and Performance programmes, then please get in touch via my website:

www.strongerself.global

If you would like to find out more about what people are doing in the world of peak performance and how they are using the tools and techniques in this book to enhance their personal and professional lives, then come across to our online community:

www.strongerself.community

Myself and my team curate special content for the community and I run a weekly webinar to deep dive into topics, techniques and strategies with a private questions and answers session. I'd love to see you there.

ACKNOWLEDGEMENTS

Writing this book has been one of the biggest challenges that I have ever faced, mentally and emotionally. I wouldn't have been able to do it if it wasn't for the resilience that I'd built in my early life and the opportunities that it has given me.

I want to thank both of my parents for always supporting me in everything I do, and they've done so much for me I can't list it all here, but some things that stand out are:

- ∞ Taking me to Judo for the first time so that I could find my own way in life.

- ∞ Buying me my first PC, a 386DX, which sparked my interest in computers.

- ∞ Funding me through university. I was the first person in my immediate family to go, and I'm immensely grateful for the opportunity. I still owe them the cruise I promised them. Dad, you'll hate a cruise ship anyway.

I'd also like to thank Peter Willment for his judo coaching at Afan Lido Judo Club and helping me to transition from junior into youth judo, and being with me as I transitioned from winning no fights to becoming Welsh Champion and gaining my black belt at seventeen.

To Laura, who is always there for me. I feel more gratitude than you could ever know. Whenever I call upon your help, you drop everything and are there for me in an instant, which gives me so much strength. You are such a great and supportive sister.

Thanks to Dave Asprey, the founder of Bulletproof®, as I would not be on this journey without your blog, podcasts and content. You and your team are delivering an important message to the world. I'd also like to give thanks to Dr Mark, Rod, Ronit and Val at the Human Potential Institute who have skilfully guided me through my coaching certifications.

I'm very grateful to Louise Papadopoullos for coaching me through this mammoth project, and for always giving me a fresh perspective and helping me when I got seriously stuck.

Thank you Liz Smallbone, my first employee, for your assistance and always being at the end of the phone when I need you. I couldn't have done what I've done in the last year without your help.

Finally, thank you to my beautiful wife Anna and my son, Rhys for their support and understanding as I've taken on this project. You've both been patient and understanding as I've closed out this project. The love you both show me every day brings so much joy to my life. You're both my world.

THE AUTHOR

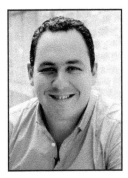

Nick is the founder of Stronger Self®. He is a specialist in human optimisation and performance and works with high-achieving entrepreneurs and senior leaders to enable them to put themselves first and take their personal and business performance to the next level.

Nick's approach has been scientifically proven using cutting-edge tools and techniques from the worlds of productivity, anti-ageing, biohacking and neuroscience, and thereby harnessing the exciting intersection between biology and technology.

Nick is a certified coach by one of the world's leading human performance organisations, the Human Potential Institute.

www.strongerself.global

www.linkedin.com/in/nickpowell

Join Nick's online community focused on increasing your performance and living a long and high-quality life:

www.strongerself.community

Lightning Source UK Ltd.
Milton Keynes UK
UKHW021751090419
340750UK00007B/387/P